Chapter 1: The Science of Strength Training

Strength training is more than just lifting weights; it's a systematic approach to enhancing the body's power, resilience, and functionality. Whether you're looking to improve athletic performance, increase muscle mass, or simply become stronger in daily life, understanding the science behind strength training is crucial for achieving long-term success. This chapter will delve into the physiological and biomechanical principles that drive strength gains, how progressive overload works, and why recovery and nutrition are indispensable components of any strength-building program.

Understanding Muscle Physiology and Biomechanics

At its core, strength training focuses on the development of muscle fibers through resistance. When you lift weights or perform other forms of resistance exercise, the muscles experience microtears, which then repair and grow back stronger. This process is known as **muscle hypertrophy**. To understand how this works, it's helpful to break down the key elements involved in muscle physiology:

- **Muscle Fibers**: Human muscles are made up of two main types of fibers: Type I (slow-twitch) and Type II (fast-twitch). Type I fibers are more endurance-oriented and are used for lighter, repetitive movements, while Type II fibers are larger and more powerful, recruited during intense, explosive efforts like heavy lifting. Strength training predominantly targets Type II fibers, which grow larger in response to heavy load and high-intensity training.
- **Muscle Contraction**: When lifting weights, the muscles contract as a result of signals from the brain. This contraction happens through the interaction of actin and myosin filaments within muscle cells. The more forcefully these filaments interact, the greater the contraction—and ultimately the stronger the muscle. Training with progressively heavier loads stimulates the muscle fibers to adapt, creating a stronger, more efficient muscle.
- **Biomechanics**: The science of movement, or biomechanics, plays a critical role in strength training. Understanding the optimal angles, joint mechanics, and body positioning during lifts ensures maximum force production while minimizing injury risk. Proper alignment and efficient movement patterns ensure that the targeted muscles are activated, and unnecessary stress is not placed on the joints.

For example, when performing a **bench press**, the shoulder blades should be retracted and depressed to create a stable base for pressing the barbell. This minimizes stress on the shoulder joints and maximizes power generation through the chest, shoulders, and triceps.

Progressive Overload Principles

Progressive overload is the cornerstone of any strength training program. This principle dictates that in order to continue making strength gains, you must gradually increase the intensity of your workouts. Without progressive overload, your body will adapt to the same stress levels, and progress will plateau. There are several ways to apply this principle:

1. **Increase Weight**: The most straightforward way to progressively overload is by increasing the amount of weight you lift. If you bench press 135 pounds for 8 reps today, your goal might be to lift 145 pounds for the same number of reps next week. Gradually adding more weight forces your muscles to handle greater stress, resulting in growth.

2. **Increase Reps or Sets**: Another form of progressive overload involves increasing the number of repetitions or sets you perform at a given weight. If you bench press 135 pounds for 8 reps today, try for 10 reps the next time. The additional volume stresses the muscle fibers further, leading to growth.

3. **Increase Training Frequency**: By training a particular muscle group more frequently, you can push your body to adapt quicker. For example, if you're training chest once per week, you might try training it twice a week, focusing on different variations of the bench press to target different aspects of the chest.

4. **Manipulate Tempo**: Slowing down the tempo (the speed at which you lift and lower the weight) increases the time under tension, which can enhance strength gains. Performing a bench press with a 3-second descent and a 1-second ascent increases muscle fatigue, leading to hypertrophy.

5. **Focus on Form and Execution**: Another critical aspect of progressive overload is improving the quality of your lifts. Each time you perfect your technique—whether it's a more controlled movement or ensuring full range of motion—you are effectively increasing the intensity, even without changing the weight.

No matter which method you use, the key is to make incremental changes. Small, consistent progress is much more sustainable in the long term than trying to make huge leaps all at once. The body responds well to gradual increases in intensity, which is why programs based on progressive overload often yield the best results.

The Role of Nutrition and Recovery in Strength Building

While exercise is the stimulus for muscle growth, **nutrition** and **recovery** are what enable muscle adaptation and growth to actually take place.

Nutrition

Carbohydrates are the body's primary energy source during high-intensity training. Consuming enough carbs ensures that the muscles have enough glycogen (stored energy) for your lifts. Healthy fats are essential for hormone production, including testosterone, which plays a significant role in muscle growth.

Hydration is equally important. Dehydration can hinder performance, decrease strength output, and increase the risk of injury. Be sure to drink enough water throughout the day to maintain peak performance.

Recovery

In addition to sleep, **active recovery** such as light stretching, foam rolling, and mobility exercises can improve circulation and reduce muscle soreness. It's essential to strike a balance between hard training and sufficient rest to prevent overtraining, which can lead to burnout and injury.

The Importance of Mastering Foundational Lifts

While strength training encompasses a wide variety of exercises, the **bench press**, **military press**, and **bent-over row** are foundational lifts that recruit multiple muscle groups and build total-body strength. Mastering these three exercises forms the basis for a well-rounded strength program.

The bench press primarily targets the chest, shoulders, and triceps. The military press emphasizes the shoulders, triceps, and upper chest, while the bent-over row focuses on the back, particularly the lats, traps, and rhomboids. Each of these movements, when executed correctly, engages the core and stabilizing muscles, providing a functional strength base that improves overall athleticism and enhances performance in everyday activities.

By mastering these lifts, you can develop raw strength and enhance functional power, which transfers to a wide range of other exercises and physical activities. Furthermore, because these lifts are compound movements, they also allow for significant load progression, making them ideal for continued muscle growth and strength.

Setting Goals and Tracking Progress

The key to success in strength training, as with any endeavor, is goal setting. Without clear objectives, it's easy to lose motivation or veer off track. Start by setting both **short-term** and **long-term** goals. A short-term goal might be to add 5 pounds to your bench press in the next month, while a long-term goal could be to bench press twice your body weight within the next year.

Tracking progress is just as essential as setting goals. Documenting the weights you lift, the number of sets and reps, and any changes in technique helps to provide measurable data on your progress. Apps or training journals are useful tools for tracking performance and ensuring that you're consistently pushing yourself to improve.

Remember that progress is not always linear. You will encounter plateaus and setbacks, but with patience and consistency, strength gains will come. The key is to stay focused on the process, adjust when necessary, and always look for ways to improve.

Conclusion

In this chapter, we've covered the foundational principles behind strength training, focusing on muscle physiology, progressive overload, and the importance of recovery and nutrition. Mastering the bench press, military press, and bent-over rows relies on understanding these core principles, as they provide the basis for achieving maximum strength. By integrating these scientific principles into your training program, you set yourself up for success and lasting gains. In the next chapter, we will explore the equipment needed to perform these exercises safely and effectively.

Chapter 2: Equipment 101

In the world of strength training, the right equipment can make all the difference between achieving optimal results and risking injury. Whether you're working out at a gym or setting up your home gym, understanding the essential equipment used for foundational lifts like the **bench press**, **military press**, and **bent-over rows** is crucial to ensure safety, efficiency, and progression. This chapter will cover the different types of equipment needed for these exercises, how to properly set them up for safe and effective lifts, and how to choose the right weights to match your strength level and training goals.

The Bench Press Apparatus

The **bench press** is one of the most iconic strength training exercises, known for building upper body power. It requires a bench and a barbell, but several considerations need to be made to ensure that you're lifting safely and effectively.

- **Flat Bench**: The flat bench is the standard for bench pressing. It provides a stable surface for you to lie on while pressing the barbell up and down. It's essential that the bench is sturdy and well-constructed to handle heavy loads without wobbling. Look for benches with adjustable heights or incline settings if you plan to experiment with different angles, such as incline or decline bench presses.
- **Barbell**: The **barbell** is the main tool used in the bench press. Standard barbells typically weigh 20 kg (44 lbs), though variations exist for lighter or heavier lifting. The barbell should have knurling (textured grips) on the shaft to provide a secure grip for your hands, especially when lifting heavy. Be sure that the barbell you use is in good condition and free from rust or damage.
- **Weight Plates**: To load the barbell with the desired resistance, you will need weight plates. These can come in a variety of materials, from rubber-coated to steel, and they typically range from 1.25 kg (2.5 lbs) to 45 kg (100 lbs). Select plates that fit securely on the barbell and ensure that they are evenly distributed to maintain balance.
- **Collars/Clamps**: These are used to secure the weight plates onto the barbell. While it's easy to overlook, collars are vital for safety, especially when using heavy weights. Without them, the plates could shift or even slide off, leading to accidents. Ensure your collars are tight enough to hold the plates in place without moving during the lift.

- **Power Rack (Optional)**: A **power rack** is highly recommended for bench pressing, especially when lifting heavy loads. It allows you to perform the exercise safely without a spotter. The rack should have adjustable safety bars set at a height where the barbell will rest if you fail the lift. This feature is crucial for avoiding injuries, as it provides a safety net in case you cannot complete the rep.

The Military Press Setup

The **military press** (also known as the overhead press) is a classic exercise for building shoulder strength and stability. The setup is slightly different from the bench press, as it requires overhead motion, but the equipment used is similar.

- **Barbell and Weight Plates**: Just like the bench press, the military press requires a barbell and weight plates. In most cases, you can use the same barbell you would for the bench press, as long as it is loaded with the appropriate weight for your training goals.
- **Rack or Squat Rack**: Unlike the bench press, the military press begins from a standing position with the barbell lifted to shoulder height. The **squat rack** or **power rack** is used to elevate the barbell at a height that allows you to lift it into position. Make sure the rack is sturdy and that the bar is set at the correct height for your body. It's important that the bar is at chest or shoulder level so that you can lift it safely without straining your back or shoulders.
- **Adjustable Bench (Optional)**: While not essential, an **adjustable bench** can be used to add an incline or decline angle to your press, shifting the emphasis slightly onto different parts of the shoulder or upper chest. It's crucial that any bench you use for the military press is stable and securely locked into place.
- **Spotter**: In some cases, a spotter may be necessary, particularly when lifting heavy overhead. A good spotter will be able to assist you if you encounter difficulty with a lift, helping to avoid any risk of dropping the barbell onto your head or shoulders.

The Bent-Over Row Setup

The **bent-over row** is a pulling exercise designed to strengthen the back, shoulders, and arms. It's typically performed using a barbell, dumbbells, or machines, but the setup for free-weight bent-over rows requires specific attention to form and safety.

- **Barbell or Dumbbells**: For the **barbell bent-over row**, the setup is very similar to that of the bench press or military press. The barbell should be loaded with the appropriate weight, and you should stand with your feet hip-width apart to maintain balance while pulling. The **dumbbell bent-over row** allows for a more unilateral approach, where you lift each arm individually, which can help correct muscle imbalances.

- **Weight Plates**: Similar to the bench press, the bent-over row uses weight plates to load the barbell. It's important that the plates are securely fastened with collars to prevent them from sliding off as you pull.

- **Platform or Weight Bench (Optional)**: While the bent-over row can be done from the floor, using a weight bench or a platform for support can provide a more controlled range of motion and reduce strain on your lower back. In a standing row, maintain a slight bend at the knees and focus on hinging at the hips, keeping your chest high and back straight to protect your spine.

- **T-Bar Row (Optional)**: For a variation of the bent-over row, the **T-bar row** is often used to isolate the back muscles with a different grip and angle. This variation requires a T-bar machine or a landmine attachment, which can provide a different type of resistance.

Proper Form and Setup for Safety

Setting up for any exercise is just as important as performing the movement itself. Proper form is critical not only for maximizing performance but also for preventing injury.

- **Bench Press Setup**: To set up for the bench press, lie flat on the bench with your feet planted firmly on the floor. Your eyes should be directly under the bar. Grip the bar slightly wider than shoulder-width, ensuring your wrists are straight and aligned with your elbows. Lower the bar slowly to your chest, maintaining control, and press it back up to the starting position. Engage your core throughout the movement, and avoid letting your feet leave the floor or arching your back excessively.
- **Military Press Setup**: Before you begin the military press, stand with the barbell positioned at shoulder height, either in a squat rack or by lifting it off the floor. Grip the barbell just outside shoulder-width with your elbows slightly in front of the bar. Engage your core and press the bar overhead in a straight line, keeping your body in a stable, upright position. Avoid leaning back or overextending your lower back, which can lead to injury.
- **Bent-Over Row Setup**: To perform the bent-over row, stand with your feet shoulder-width apart and hinge at the hips, keeping your back flat and chest up. Grip the barbell with a pronated (overhand) grip and pull the barbell towards your lower chest or upper abdomen, ensuring that your elbows stay close to your body. Keep your core engaged throughout the movement to protect your spine from excessive strain.

Choosing the Right Weights and Adjusting for Progress

Selecting the right weights for each exercise is crucial to ensure you are challenging your muscles without overloading them, which can lead to injury.

- **Starting Light**: If you're new to strength training or a particular exercise, it's important to start light. Mastering the technique should be your primary focus before adding weight. Lifting too heavy too soon can compromise your form and increase the risk of injury.
- **Progressing Gradually**: As you gain strength, you can gradually increase the weight. Aim for a weight that allows you to perform the exercise with good form while still being challenging. For compound exercises like the bench press and military press, aim for sets of 6-12 reps, which is a range that promotes both strength and hypertrophy.
- **Adjusting for Plateaus**: If you hit a plateau and aren't making progress, it may be time to adjust the weights or use progressive techniques like tempo manipulation or incorporating accessory movements to strengthen weak points.

Conclusion

The right equipment, proper setup, and correct form are the cornerstones of a successful strength training program. By understanding how to use the bench press, military press, and bent-over row apparatus safely and effectively, you're setting yourself up for success in building total-body strength. As you progress, remember that selecting the appropriate weights and maintaining safety should always be your priority. In the next chapter, we will explore the core movements of these exercises and how they fit into a well-rounded strength training regimen.

Chapter 3: Understanding the Core Movements

In strength training, the **bench press**, **military press**, and **bent-over rows** are three of the most effective compound exercises for building upper-body strength and overall athletic performance. These foundational lifts are integral to a full-body workout because they target multiple muscle groups simultaneously, engage stabilizing muscles, and promote functional strength. This chapter will explore how these core movements fit into a complete training regimen, the muscles they target, and the importance of complementary accessory exercises to enhance your strength and prevent imbalances.

The Bench Press: Targeting the Chest, Shoulders, and Triceps

The **bench press** is widely regarded as the gold standard for building upper body pushing strength. Its main muscles targeted are the **pectoralis major** (chest), **deltoids** (shoulders), and **triceps brachii** (arms). However, the bench press also engages a range of secondary muscles that contribute to stability and control.

Primary Muscles

- **Pectoralis Major**: The chest muscles are the prime movers in the bench press, especially the sternal part of the pectoralis major. The wider the grip, the more the chest is emphasized.
- **Deltoids (Shoulders)**: The anterior deltoids (front part of the shoulders) work to stabilize the bar and assist with the press.
- **Triceps**: The triceps play a crucial role in locking out the bar at the top of the movement and are heavily involved during the final portion of the press.

Secondary Muscles

- **Serratus Anterior:** The muscles on the sides of the rib cage help with the stabilization of the scapulae, especially during the lowering phase of the lift.
- **Rhomboids and Trapezius:** These upper back muscles stabilize the shoulder blades, keeping them retracted and preventing shoulder injury.
- **Core:** A strong core is essential for maintaining proper body position on the bench, especially when lifting heavy.

How it fits into a full-body workout:

The bench press is a **compound exercise**, meaning it works several large muscle groups at once. It can be performed on a dedicated upper-body day or integrated into a full-body workout routine. The bench press complements other pressing movements, such as the **military press**, and pulling exercises like the **bent-over row**, balancing push-pull dynamics for optimal strength development.

The Military Press: Strengthening Shoulders and Triceps

The **military press** (or overhead press) is a fundamental overhead pressing movement that strengthens the shoulders, upper chest, and triceps, while also engaging the core and stabilizer muscles.

Primary Muscles

- **Deltoids**: The military press targets all three heads of the deltoids, with a particular emphasis on the anterior and medial (front and middle) deltoid muscles.
- **Triceps**: The triceps assist with the pressing motion and help extend the elbows, especially as the bar is locked overhead.
- **Upper Chest**: The upper portion of the pectoralis major is involved in the lift, especially when pressing at slightly forward angles.

Secondary Muscles

- **Upper Back**: The trapezius and rhomboids stabilize the shoulders and neck region, ensuring control during the lift.
- **Core**: The core muscles (rectus abdominis, obliques, and lower back) must engage to maintain stability and prevent excessive lower back arching, particularly when the weight is heavy.
- **Forearms and Grip**: Grip strength and forearm stability are essential for controlling the barbell overhead.

How it fits into a full-body workout:

The military press can be performed as a standalone lift on shoulder or upper-body days. It works synergistically with other pressing movements, like the bench press, and pulling movements, such as the bent-over row, to create a well-rounded upper-body workout. The vertical press pattern of the military press contrasts with the horizontal push of the bench press, offering variety for shoulder development and functional strength.

The Bent-Over Row: Building the Back and Strengthening the Posterior Chain

The **bent-over row** is a classic pulling exercise that targets the **posterior chain** (the muscles along the back of the body), including the lats, rhomboids, traps, and lower back. It is a key exercise for building strength and mass in the back, balancing out the pushing movements of the bench press and military press.

Primary Muscles

- **Latissimus Dorsi**: The lats are the main muscles worked in the bent-over row, responsible for pulling the arms downward and inward. They are essential for creating a V-shaped back.
- **Rhomboids**: Located between the shoulder blades, the rhomboids retract the scapulae, pulling them toward the spine. This helps with shoulder stability and posture.
- **Trapezius**: The traps assist in scapular retraction and shoulder stability. The middle and lower parts of the traps are engaged when pulling the barbell toward the torso.

Secondary Muscles

- **Biceps**: While the biceps are secondary muscles in the bent-over row, they assist with elbow flexion and control the bar as you pull.
- **Posterior Deltoids**: The rear delts help stabilize the shoulders during the row and assist in the movement, especially when pulling with heavier loads.
- **Core**: Like the military press, the core plays a significant role in stabilizing the body and maintaining a neutral spine throughout the row. Proper engagement of the abs and lower back is critical to prevent injury.

How it fits into a full-body workout:

The bent-over row is an excellent pulling exercise that should be incorporated into any upper-body workout, especially on back or pulling-focused days. It balances out the pushing exercises, ensuring that both the anterior and posterior parts of the upper body are trained effectively. Incorporating rows into your routine enhances upper back strength, posture, and scapular mobility, making it a vital exercise for functional movement.

The Importance of Accessory Exercises

While the bench press, military press, and bent-over row form the core of a strength program, **accessory exercises** are equally important for addressing muscle imbalances, strengthening weak points, and improving overall movement patterns.

For the Bench Press

- **Tricep Dips**: Dips are a great accessory movement to strengthen the triceps, helping with the lockout phase of the bench press.
- **Rotator Cuff Exercises**: Strengthening the rotator cuff muscles is crucial for shoulder health and injury prevention. External rotations and band pull-aparts are effective exercises.
- **Chest Flys**: These isolate the chest muscles and can help develop more muscle mass in the pectorals, complementing the press.

For the Military Press

- **Lateral Raises**: These target the middle deltoid and can help balance out shoulder development for improved pressing strength.
- **Face Pulls**: This exercise targets the rear deltoids and upper traps, enhancing shoulder stability and posture.
- **Shrugs**: Shrugging helps build trap strength, which contributes to shoulder stability during the press.

For the Bent-Over Row

- **Pull-Ups/Chin-Ups**: These are excellent bodyweight exercises for developing the back muscles, particularly the lats and biceps.
- **Single-Arm Dumbbell Rows**: This exercise isolates each side of the back and helps correct muscle imbalances.
- **Back Extensions**: Strengthening the lower back is crucial for maintaining proper posture and spinal alignment during rowing movements.

Integrating the Core Movements into a Full-Body Workout Routine

When building a full-body workout, it's essential to strategically integrate these core lifts with accessory exercises for a balanced approach. A typical weekly strength training program may look like this:

Day 1 (Upper Body Push/Pull)

- Bench Press (4 sets of 6-8 reps)
- Military Press (3 sets of 6-8 reps)
- Bent-Over Rows (4 sets of 6-8 reps)
- Accessory: Tricep Dips, Pull-Ups

Day 2 (Lower Body/Core)

- Squats, Deadlifts, Lunges
- Core Work (Planks, Leg Raises)

Day 3 (Upper Body Push/Pull)

- Bench Press (4 sets of 6-8 reps)
- Military Press (3 sets of 6-8 reps)
- Accessory: Lateral Raises, Face Pulls, Shrugs

Day 4 (Active Recovery)

Mobility Work, Stretching, Light Cardio

Conclusion

Understanding how the bench press, military press, and bent-over row fit into a full-body workout is key to structuring an effective and balanced strength training routine. These compound exercises target large muscle groups and work synergistically to promote total-body strength and functional fitness. Complementing them with accessory movements ensures that you develop all the muscles needed for powerful and injury-free performance. In the next chapter, we will dive deeper into common mistakes and how to avoid them, so you can perfect your form and continue to progress safely and effectively.

Chapter 4: Common Mistakes and How to Avoid Them

In any strength training journey, understanding the correct technique for the bench press, military press, and bent-over row is crucial for long-term progress and injury prevention. Despite their effectiveness, these exercises are often performed incorrectly, leading to suboptimal results or, worse, injuries. This chapter will explore the most common mistakes made during these three foundational lifts and provide corrective techniques to enhance performance, prevent injury, and ensure consistent gains. Whether you're a beginner or an experienced lifter, mastering form is the key to maximizing strength.

Common Mistakes in the Bench Press

The bench press is one of the most widely performed exercises, but it's also one of the most prone to mistakes. Here are the key errors often seen in the bench press and how to correct them:

Incorrect Bar Path

- **Mistake**: Letting the bar drift forward or down towards the neck rather than following a straight line.
- **Correction**: The bar should travel in a slightly diagonal path, coming down to your mid-chest. This helps ensure maximum chest activation and reduces strain on the shoulders.

Feet Off the Floor

- **Mistake**: Lifting your feet off the floor or placing them on the bench.
- **Correction**: Keep your feet planted firmly on the floor to provide stability and activate your legs. This creates a solid base for generating force and maintaining body alignment.

Elbows Flaring Out Too Much

- **Mistake**: Letting your elbows flare out at a 90-degree angle from your body.
- **Correction**: Aim to keep your elbows at about a 45-degree angle to your torso. This will keep the shoulders in a safer position and improve pressing power.

Lifting Your Hips Off the Bench

- **Mistake**: Arching your lower back too excessively, leading to the hips lifting off the bench.
- **Correction**: Maintain a neutral spine throughout the lift, ensuring that only your chest and feet are in contact with the bench. A slight arch in the lower back is fine, but avoid excessive lumbar extension.

Not Engaging the Lats

- **Mistake**: Failing to activate the lats during the lowering phase of the bench press.
- **Correction**: Before you press, engage your lats by squeezing them down and back. This helps with stability, keeps your shoulders protected, and improves overall pressing power.

Bouncing the Bar Off the Chest

- **Mistake**: Letting the bar bounce off the chest in an effort to use momentum for the lift.
- **Correction**: Lower the bar under control and pause for a brief moment before pressing it back up. This ensures full muscle activation and minimizes the risk of injury.

Common Mistakes in the Military Press

The military press is an essential lift for shoulder and upper body development, but it requires precision to execute correctly. Common errors include:

Overarching the Lower Back

- **Mistake**: Using excessive lower back arching to press the bar overhead, which can strain the spine.
- **Correction**: Engage your core and squeeze your glutes to prevent arching. Maintain a neutral spine throughout the press to protect your lower back.

Elbows Flaring Too Much

- **Mistake**: Flailing the elbows out excessively during the press.
- **Correction**: Keep the elbows slightly in front of the bar to minimize shoulder strain. The bar should follow a vertical path rather than a forward arc.

Pressing Too Far Behind the Head

- **Mistake**: Pressing the bar too far behind the head, often resulting in shoulder discomfort.
- **Correction**: Press the bar directly overhead, staying in line with the ears. This helps keep the shoulder joints in a safer, more stable position.

Not Engaging the Core

- **Mistake**: Failing to engage the core, which leads to instability and poor posture.
- **Correction**: Brace your core tightly before initiating the press. This provides support for your spine and helps maintain a stable torso throughout the movement.

Relying Too Much on the Legs

- **Mistake**: Using excessive leg drive to assist with the press, turning the movement into a push press.
- **Correction**: The military press should be performed with minimal leg involvement. Only engage the legs if you're performing a push press or jerk variation. Focus on pressing with the shoulders and arms.

Common Mistakes in the Bent-Over Row

The bent-over row is an excellent pulling movement, but it can lead to imbalances or back issues if not performed correctly. Here are common errors and how to fix them:

Rounded Back

- **Mistake**: Allowing the back to round during the rowing motion, which places undue stress on the spine and increases the risk of injury.
- **Correction**: Maintain a neutral spine by engaging your core and pulling your shoulder blades back. A slight bend in the knees is acceptable, but the back should stay straight throughout the movement.

Using Too Much Weight

- **Mistake**: Lifting a weight that's too heavy, resulting in a lack of control and improper form.
- **Correction**: Choose a weight that allows you to control the movement with a full range of motion. Focus on controlled movements rather than attempting to lift as much as possible.

Not Retracting the Scapula

- **Mistake**: Failing to engage the upper back by not retracting the shoulder blades during the row.
- **Correction**: Initiate the movement by pulling the shoulder blades back and down before bending your elbows. This engages the upper back muscles more effectively and protects the shoulders.

Pulling the Elbows Too High

- **Mistake**: Lifting the elbows too high, which shifts the focus to the traps and reduces activation of the lats.
- **Correction**: Keep the elbows at a 45-degree angle to your torso, aiming to keep them close to the body as you row. This engages the lats more effectively.

Jerking or Using Momentum

- **Mistake**: Using momentum to swing the weight rather than engaging the muscles in a controlled fashion.
- **Correction**: Perform the movement slowly and deliberately, ensuring each rep is controlled. Focus on squeezing the muscles at the top of the movement before lowering the weight.

Preventing Injuries and Long-Term Issues

Mastering proper technique not only improves strength but also plays a critical role in preventing injury. Here are some general tips to safeguard your body during strength training:

1. **Warm-Up Properly**: Always perform a dynamic warm-up before lifting to prepare your muscles, joints, and nervous system for the work ahead. Focus on the muscle groups you'll be training and include mobility exercises for the shoulders, hips, and back.

2. **Use Full Range of Motion**: Avoid cutting the range of motion short, which can lead to muscular imbalances. For example, in the bench press, ensure that the bar touches your chest each time, and in rows, aim for a full retraction of the scapula.

3. **Progress Gradually**: Progressive overload is crucial, but adding weight too quickly can cause injuries. Increase weight by small increments and focus on maintaining form rather than lifting heavy weight prematurely.

4. **Listen to Your Body**: Pay attention to any discomfort or pain. It's normal to feel muscle fatigue, but sharp or persistent pain can be a sign of overuse or poor form. Always back off if you feel something isn't right.

5. **Prioritize Recovery**: Strength training puts significant stress on your muscles and joints, so recovery is just as important as the lifting itself. Ensure you're getting enough rest, proper nutrition, and stretching to maintain flexibility and muscle health.

Conclusion

Avoiding common mistakes in the bench press, military press, and bent-over row is crucial for building strength, improving performance, and preventing injury. By focusing on proper form, listening to your body, and implementing corrective techniques, you'll be able to progress efficiently and safely in your strength training journey. In the next chapter, we'll explore how to structure your workout program to maximize results and incorporate these movements for long-term success.

Chapter 5: How to Structure Your Program

Designing a strength training program is an essential step in your journey toward mastery of the bench press, military press, and bent-over rows. Whether you're a beginner or an advanced lifter, structuring a program effectively will ensure that you develop strength, enhance performance, and avoid plateaus. This chapter provides a guide for creating a balanced workout plan that aligns with your goals, fitness level, and desired outcomes.

Designing a Balanced Workout Plan

A well-structured strength training program focuses on progressively increasing load and intensity while maintaining balance across muscle groups. Here's how to design a program that will effectively target all the muscles involved in the bench press, military press, and bent-over row:

Establish Your Goals

- **Strength Focus**: If your goal is to maximize strength, prioritize compound movements (bench press, military press, and bent-over rows) with low-to-moderate reps (3-6 per set) and high intensity. Focus on lifting progressively heavier weights while maintaining proper form.
- **Hypertrophy Focus**: If muscle growth is the goal, work in the 6-12 rep range with moderate to heavy weights. Incorporate accessory exercises and increase volume to target muscle fatigue and stimulate muscle growth.
- **Endurance Focus**: If endurance is your goal, aim for higher reps (12-20 per set) with lighter weights, incorporating techniques like supersets or circuit training to improve muscular stamina.

Program Frequency

Beginners

- Day 1: Bench press, military press, accessory shoulder and chest exercises.
- Day 2: Bent-over row, accessory back and arm exercises.
- Day 3: Compound lifts (lower body or full body with moderate-intensity variations).

- **Intermediate Lifters**: Aim for 4-5 training days per week. A typical program may include a push-pull split (e.g., upper body push/upper body pull/lower body) to allow sufficient recovery while increasing training volume and intensity.
- **Advanced Lifters**: 5-6 days per week, incorporating specialized programs like push-pull-legs, or periodized programs that cycle intensity and volume across weeks to maximize strength and hypertrophy.

Volume and Intensity

- **Strength Focus**: Use lower volume but high intensity. This means fewer sets (3-5 sets) with low reps (3-6 reps) at higher intensities (80-90% of your 1RM).
- **Hypertrophy Focus**: Moderate intensity and volume. Perform 4-6 sets of 6-12 reps, working with weights that are around 70-80% of your 1RM.
- **Endurance Focus**: High volume, moderate-to-low intensity. Aim for 3-5 sets of 12-20 reps with lighter weights (50-70% of your 1RM).

Progressive Overload

- **Increase Weight**: Gradually increase the weight lifted each week or every other week.
- **Increase Reps or Sets**: Start with a moderate weight and gradually increase the number of reps or sets you perform.
- **Adjust Tempo**: Slow down the eccentric (lowering) phase of the lift to increase time under tension, or use a pause at the bottom of the lift to build strength and stability.

Combining Compound and Isolation Exercises

While the bench press, military press, and bent-over rows are essential compound lifts that target multiple muscle groups, accessory exercises can complement them by focusing on specific muscles, preventing imbalances, and improving your performance. Here's how to structure your program:

Primary Compound Movements

- **Bench Press**: Target chest, shoulders, and triceps.
- **Military Press**: Focus on shoulders, triceps, and upper chest.
- **Bent-Over Row**: Target the back, traps, biceps, and rear delts.

Accessory Movements

- **Chest and Shoulders**: Dumbbell presses, chest flyes, lateral raises, front raises.
- **Back and Biceps**: Lat pulldowns, dumbbell rows, barbell curls, face pulls.
- **Triceps and Forearms**: Tricep dips, tricep pushdowns, wrist curls.

3. These exercises not only help build muscle and increase strength but also protect the joints and tendons involved in the primary lifts, reducing the risk of injury and overuse.

4. **Core Training**

    A strong core is vital for stability and posture during all strength movements. Incorporate core exercises like planks, Russian twists, leg raises, and cable woodchoppers to build functional strength and improve overall lifting technique.

Frequency, Volume, and Intensity Recommendations

The frequency, volume, and intensity of your program will vary based on your level and goals. Here's how to apply these principles to different stages of lifting:

For Beginners

- **Frequency**: 3-4 days per week.
- **Volume**: Moderate (3-4 sets per exercise, 8-12 reps).
- **Intensity**: Moderate (50-70% of 1RM).
- **Program Structure**: Full-body workouts, focusing on basic form and building endurance.

For Intermediate Lifters

- **Frequency**: 4-5 days per week.
- **Volume**: Higher (4-6 sets per exercise, 6-10 reps).
- **Intensity**: Moderate to heavy (70-85% of 1RM).
- **Program Structure**: Split programs like push/pull/legs, with accessory exercises to target weak points.

For Advanced Lifters

- **Frequency**: 5-6 days per week.
- **Volume**: Very high (4-8 sets per exercise, 3-6 reps for strength, 6-12 reps for hypertrophy).
- **Intensity**: Heavy (85-95% of 1RM).
- **Program Structure**: Periodized programs with varying intensity and volume, along with advanced techniques like supersets, drop sets, and training to failure.

Tracking Progress

Tracking your progress is essential to measure improvements and make necessary adjustments to your training program. Use the following strategies to stay on top of your strength gains:

1. **Log Your Lifts**: Keep a workout journal or use an app to track the weights, sets, and reps for each exercise. This will help you see when it's time to increase the load or change your program.
2. **Assess Strength Gains**: Track improvements in key lifts (bench press, military press, and bent-over rows). Periodically test your 1RM to measure overall progress.
3. **Monitor Recovery**: Record how well you recover after each workout. If you're consistently feeling fatigued or noticing declining performance, it may be time to adjust your intensity or recovery strategies.
4. **Set Milestones**: Break down larger goals into smaller, manageable milestones. For example, instead of aiming for a 100-pound bench press increase, set smaller incremental goals like increasing your 5-rep max by 5 pounds each month.

Conclusion

A well-structured program is the foundation of your strength training journey. By combining the bench press, military press, and bent-over rows with accessory exercises, managing frequency, volume, and intensity, and tracking your progress, you'll be on the path to strength mastery. In the following chapters, we'll dive deeper into each of these lifts, providing specific techniques, variations, and strategies to help you reach new levels of power and performance.

Chapter 6: The Bench Press: Overview and Benefits

The bench press is often considered the cornerstone of upper body strength training. This classic lift has earned its place as a fundamental exercise in powerlifting, bodybuilding, and general strength programs. In this chapter, we'll delve into the anatomy of the bench press, explore its benefits, and discuss how mastering this movement can lead to impressive gains in both strength and muscle development.

Anatomy of the Bench Press

The bench press is a compound movement, meaning it recruits multiple muscle groups simultaneously. Its primary muscles involved are:

1. **Pectoralis Major**: The chest muscles are the main drivers during the press. The bench press effectively targets the clavicular (upper) and sternal (middle and lower) portions of the chest, making it a powerful exercise for overall chest development.
2. **Deltoids**: The shoulders, particularly the anterior (front) deltoids, assist in pressing the barbell away from the chest. They stabilize the movement and help initiate the press, contributing to overall shoulder strength.
3. **Triceps Brachii**: The triceps play a crucial role in locking out the elbows at the top of the press. As you push the bar upward, the triceps work to extend your arms, contributing to the power needed for the lift.
4. **Rhomboids and Trapezius**: While the rhomboids and traps aren't the primary movers, they provide stabilization through the scapular retraction process, helping ensure a strong and safe press.
5. **Serratus Anterior**: This muscle, which helps protract the scapula, assists in the movement by keeping the shoulder blade stable and supporting the pressing motion.

Understanding these key muscle groups helps explain why the bench press is such an effective exercise for building upper body strength. By engaging both large and small muscle groups, it maximizes overall muscular development while improving functional strength.

Key Benefits of the Bench Press

The bench press offers numerous benefits that extend beyond mere aesthetic improvement:

1. **Upper Body Strength**: One of the most obvious benefits is the increase in upper body strength. A stronger bench press translates into better performance in other lifts and daily activities, as well as increased force production for athletes involved in contact sports or explosive movements.

2. **Muscle Hypertrophy**: The bench press is an essential exercise for building chest, shoulder, and tricep size. Consistently challenging these muscle groups with progressive overload leads to hypertrophy (muscle growth) and improved muscular endurance.

3. **Functional Strength**: The motion of the bench press mimics various real-world movements, such as pushing, pressing, or lifting heavy objects. As such, mastering the bench press builds functional strength that translates into better performance in sports and physical tasks.

4. **Bone Density and Joint Health**: Regularly performing the bench press, particularly with progressive loading, can help increase bone density, particularly in the wrists, elbows, and shoulders. Additionally, the controlled range of motion helps reinforce healthy joint movement, contributing to long-term joint integrity.

5. **Improved Confidence**: The bench press is a key strength marker for many lifters. As you increase your bench press performance, you'll likely experience a boost in self-confidence, which can spill over into other areas of life.

Variations of the Bench Press

While the traditional barbell bench press is the most well-known variation, there are several other ways to perform this exercise to target muscles from different angles and provide variety to your training routine:

1. **Incline Bench Press**: Performed on an inclined bench (usually set at a 30-45-degree angle), this variation places more emphasis on the upper chest and shoulders. It's an excellent way to develop the upper portion of the pectorals and deltoids.
2. **Decline Bench Press**: This variation is performed on a declined bench, targeting the lower chest. It can be an excellent option for individuals looking to enhance the development of the sternal portion of the pectorals.
3. **Dumbbell Bench Press**: Using dumbbells instead of a barbell allows for a greater range of motion and engages more stabilizing muscles, as each arm works independently. This variation is great for correcting imbalances and increasing overall muscle activation.
4. **Close-Grip Bench Press**: By narrowing the hand placement, this variation places more emphasis on the triceps while still working the chest and shoulders. It's a great accessory movement for improving lockout strength in the bench press.
5. **Paused Bench Press**: In this variation, you pause at the bottom of the lift for 1-2 seconds before pressing the bar back up. The pause eliminates any momentum, forcing your muscles to generate maximum force from a dead stop, which increases strength at the bottom of the lift.

6. **Floor Press**: Performed lying on the floor, this variation eliminates the leg drive and reduces the range of motion, allowing you to target the triceps and chest more effectively. It is often used to improve the upper portion of the press.

The Mental Aspect of the Bench Press

The bench press is as much a mental exercise as it is a physical one. Mental preparation and focus are essential for success in the lift. Here's how to enhance your mindset for maximal performance:

1. **Visualization**: Before you approach the bench, visualize the entire lift in your mind. Picture the bar path, your breathing, and your form. Visualizing success can boost confidence and reduce performance anxiety.

2. **Focus on Breathing**: Proper breathing is crucial for maintaining intra-abdominal pressure and stabilizing your torso. Inhale deeply as you lower the bar to your chest, and exhale forcefully as you push the bar up. Establishing a rhythmic breathing pattern helps maintain focus and energy throughout the lift.

3. **Control the Tempo**: Resist the urge to rush the lift. Lower the bar in a controlled manner, allowing your muscles to work through their full range of motion. Press the bar explosively but with control to ensure proper technique and reduce the risk of injury.

4. **Positive Self-Talk**: Use affirmations and positive self-talk to push past mental barriers. Remind yourself of your strength and past achievements. A strong mental attitude can often be the difference between hitting a PR and failing a lift.

5. **Use a Spotter**: For safety and mental confidence, always use a spotter when bench pressing heavy loads. Knowing that someone is there to assist you in case of failure allows you to push harder and take more risks in your training.

Conclusion

The bench press is a powerhouse movement that targets multiple muscle groups and delivers significant strength and hypertrophy benefits. Whether you're a beginner or an advanced lifter, mastering the bench press will not only help you build a solid upper body foundation but also contribute to greater functional strength, joint health, and mental resilience. In the next chapter, we will break down the key components of perfecting your bench press form, ensuring that you lift with precision, power, and safety.

Chapter 7: Perfecting Your Form

Form is everything when it comes to strength training, especially with foundational lifts like the bench press. A slight deviation in technique can lead to inefficiencies, prevent maximum performance, and even cause injury. In this chapter, we will break down the steps to perfect your bench press form, covering everything from hand placement to bar path, foot positioning, and breathing techniques. Mastering these details will ensure you not only perform the lift safely but also unlock your full potential.

1. Hand Placement

Your hand placement on the barbell will determine the angle of the press and which muscles are activated most. Getting this right is essential for both power and safety.

- **Standard Hand Position**: For the conventional bench press, grip the barbell with your hands slightly wider than shoulder-width apart. Your forearms should be vertical when the barbell is lowered to your chest. If your hands are too narrow or too wide, you risk compromising the efficiency of the lift, affecting your chest activation, and increasing the chance of shoulder strain.
- **Grip Type**: The most common grip is the **overhand grip**, where the palms face away from you. Ensure your thumbs are wrapped securely around the bar to prevent the bar from slipping. This grip maximizes control and power.
- **Thumb Position**: The **thumb-over grip** is the safest option. The "thumbless" or "suicide" grip (thumbs not wrapped around the bar) can increase the risk of the bar slipping, especially under heavy loads. Avoid using this grip unless you have experience and are using a spotter.
- **Elbow Angle**: When your arms are fully extended at the top of the press, your elbows should be locked out but not overextended. Keep your elbows in line with your wrists throughout the lift to prevent shoulder strain.

2. Foot Positioning

Your feet provide the base of support for the entire lift. Proper foot placement stabilizes your body, engages your core, and allows for greater power transfer.

- **Feet Flat on the Ground**: Your feet should be flat on the floor with your knees bent at about a 90-degree angle. Avoid letting your feet lift off the ground during the press as this can destabilize your body and shift focus away from the target muscles.

- **Driving Through the Heels**: While pressing, think of "driving through your heels" to activate the posterior chain (glutes, hamstrings, and lower back). This engages your core, which helps keep your body rigid and prevents arching your lower back excessively.

- **Foot Placement for Stability**: You may prefer to position your feet directly beneath your knees or slightly further out to achieve maximum stability. The key is ensuring that your feet are planted firmly to avoid any instability.

- **Leg Drive**: Some lifters use leg drive to generate power and assist the press. To do this, push your feet into the ground (without lifting your heels) as you press the bar up. This should feel like you are "bridging" your body into the bar.

3. Bar Path

The bar path refers to the trajectory that the barbell follows during the press. Maintaining a proper bar path is critical for optimizing power and reducing injury risk.

- **Lowering the Bar**: When bringing the bar down to your chest, lower it to a point just below your nipples or around the sternum area. Keep your elbows at about a 45-degree angle to your body, not flaring out excessively, which can strain the shoulders.
- **Pressing the Bar**: The bar should follow a slightly curved path. As you press the bar upward, think of pushing the bar back slightly towards your head, following a natural arc. Avoid a straight line path, as this can cause unnecessary strain on your shoulders and wrists.
- **Lockout Position**: At the top of the press, your elbows should be fully extended but not hyperextended. The bar should be directly over your shoulders, with your arms perpendicular to the floor.
- **Bar Speed**: Aim for a controlled descent and an explosive ascent. The bar should descend in a controlled manner for a few seconds (around 2-3 seconds) and then explode upward, using your full body's power. This controlled lowering phase helps in muscle recruitment and reduces the risk of injury.

4. Torso Engagement and Upper Back Positioning

Maintaining a rigid torso is essential for proper technique and power during the bench press. Many lifters neglect their upper back, which can result in a lack of stability and reduced force output.

- **Retracting the Scapula**: Before you unrack the bar, squeeze your shoulder blades together and down as if you're trying to pinch a pencil between your shoulder blades. This scapular retraction helps to stabilize your upper back and create a solid platform for pressing.
- **Chest Up**: Keeping your chest proud (lifting it slightly) is crucial for proper bench press mechanics. Imagine puffing your chest out and upward. This slight chest elevation minimizes stress on the shoulder joints and helps you press more effectively.
- **Maintaining a Neutral Spine**: Your spine should remain in a neutral position throughout the lift. This means avoiding excessive arching of your lower back, which can put undue strain on your spine and lead to injury.

5. Breathing Techniques for Maximum Efficiency

Proper breathing is critical to supporting the press and maintaining control throughout the movement.

- **Inhale Before Lowering the Bar**: Before you start lowering the bar to your chest, take a deep breath and fill your lungs with air. This helps create intra-abdominal pressure, which supports your spine and torso during the lift.
- **Brace Your Core**: As you inhale, tighten your core muscles as if you're about to get punched in the stomach. This bracing creates a solid foundation for your body, preventing any instability during the press.
- **Exhale During the Push**: As you press the bar upward, exhale forcefully. This helps you to maintain focus, reduce pressure in your chest, and push with maximum force.
- **Breathing Cadence**: Find a rhythm that works for you, but generally, aim to exhale during the concentric phase (pressing the bar up) and inhale during the eccentric phase (lowering the bar).

6. Common Mistakes to Avoid

Now that we've covered the key elements of perfect form, let's quickly review some common mistakes and how to avoid them:

- **Flared Elbows**: Allowing your elbows to flare out excessively during the descent puts unnecessary stress on the shoulder joints. Instead, aim to keep your elbows at a 45-degree angle to your body.
- **Uneven Grip**: A misaligned grip on the bar can cause uneven force distribution, leading to a lopsided press. Ensure your hands are symmetrically placed, and the bar is balanced.
- **Arching the Lower Back**: Excessive lower back arching can lead to lumbar strain. Keep your back neutral and avoid overextending your spine.
- **Bouncing the Bar**: Bouncing the bar off your chest can cause serious injuries to your ribs and sternum. Always lower the bar in a controlled manner and press it back up without relying on momentum.
- **Incomplete Lockout**: Failing to fully extend your arms at the top of the lift reduces the effectiveness of the press. Ensure you reach a complete lockout at the top.

Conclusion

Mastering the bench press form takes time and attention to detail. By focusing on hand placement, foot positioning, bar path, torso engagement, and breathing, you will ensure you are lifting with maximum power and efficiency. As with all strength training movements, consistency and patience are key to making continuous progress. In the next chapter, we will explore accessory exercises that complement the bench press, helping to strengthen weak points and prevent injury.

Chapter 8: Accessory Movements for the Bench Press

While the bench press is one of the most effective exercises for building upper body strength, it is only part of the equation when it comes to achieving true power and performance. Accessory exercises play a critical role in strengthening weak points, improving overall muscle balance, and reducing the risk of injury. In this chapter, we will explore key accessory movements designed to enhance your bench press, focusing on rotator cuff strengthening, shoulder mobility, and stabilizing muscle groups.

1. Rotator Cuff Strengthening

The rotator cuff is a group of muscles and tendons that stabilize the shoulder joint, allowing for safe and effective pressing movements. Weakness or imbalances in the rotator cuff can lead to shoulder injuries, affecting both your bench press and other upper body lifts.

- **External Rotations**: One of the best exercises to target the rotator cuff is the external rotation. Using a light dumbbell or a resistance band, hold the weight at your side and rotate your arm outward, keeping your elbow tucked in at a 90-degree angle. Perform this exercise slowly and with control to ensure you're working the smaller stabilizer muscles of the shoulder.
- **Face Pulls**: A powerful accessory exercise for the rotator cuff is the face pull, which also works the rear deltoids and upper traps. Using a rope attachment on a cable machine, set the pulley at face height and pull the rope toward your face, keeping your elbows high and squeezing your shoulder blades together. This exercise improves shoulder stability and posture, both of which are crucial for a solid bench press.
- **Prone Y Raises**: Lie face down on a bench and hold light dumbbells in each hand. With your arms extended in a "Y" shape, raise your arms overhead, squeezing your shoulder blades together. This exercise targets the lower traps and helps to improve shoulder stability, which is essential for controlling the barbell during the bench press.

- **Internal Rotations**: Although external rotations are more commonly emphasized, internal rotations can also help in balancing shoulder strength. Perform these by holding a resistance band at shoulder height and rotating your arm inward across your body. This exercise complements external rotations by targeting the internal rotator muscles, contributing to overall shoulder health.

2. Shoulder Mobility

Optimal shoulder mobility is crucial for ensuring proper bench press form and avoiding shoulder strain. Limited range of motion in the shoulders can prevent you from achieving a full range of motion during the press, reducing the effectiveness of the lift and increasing the risk of injury. Here are some exercises and stretches to enhance shoulder mobility:

- **Scapular Wall Slides**: Stand with your back against a wall, your feet a few inches away from it. Press your lower back, upper back, and head into the wall, and raise your arms into a "W" shape with your elbows bent. Slowly slide your arms up the wall, aiming for the "Y" position while maintaining contact between your arms and the wall. This exercise improves scapular mobility and engages the muscles of the rotator cuff.

- **Chest Openers**: Perform chest-opening stretches by interlacing your fingers behind your back and lifting your arms upward, squeezing your shoulder blades together. This stretch opens up the chest and enhances the flexibility needed for a proper bar path on the bench press. You can also perform this stretch using a resistance band for greater activation.

- **Shoulder Dislocations (or Pass-Throughs)**: Using a resistance band or PVC pipe, hold the object with a wide grip and slowly pass it overhead, moving the shoulders through their full range of motion. This exercise is excellent for improving shoulder flexibility and preparing the shoulders for pressing movements.

- **Band Pull-Aparts**: Hold a resistance band in front of you with both hands. Keep your arms straight and pull the band apart by retracting your shoulder blades. This exercise helps activate the posterior shoulder muscles, improving shoulder mobility and stability. It's especially useful as a warm-up before heavier bench press sets.

3. Stabilizing Muscle Groups

While the primary focus of the bench press is on the chest, shoulders, and triceps, the stability of the entire upper body contributes to your overall performance. Strengthening stabilizing muscles helps prevent compensatory movements that can limit your strength and increase your injury risk.

- **Planks**: A strong core is essential for maintaining stability during the bench press. Planks engage the abdominals, lower back, and obliques, teaching your body to maintain rigidity while pressing. Adding variations such as side planks or plank reaches can further enhance core strength and stability.
- **Dead Bugs**: The dead bug is a great exercise for improving core stability and coordination. Lie on your back with your arms extended toward the ceiling and your knees bent at 90 degrees. Slowly extend one arm and the opposite leg toward the floor while keeping your lower back pressed into the ground. Return to the starting position and alternate sides. This movement teaches control of the core, which translates to better stability while pressing heavy weights.
- **Farmer's Walks**: While this exercise primarily targets grip strength, it also works the entire body, including the core, traps, and shoulders. By holding heavy dumbbells or kettlebells in each hand, walk a set distance while maintaining an upright posture. This exercise improves your ability to stabilize your torso under load, which helps keep your body rigid during the bench press.
- **Turkish Get-Ups**: This total-body exercise improves shoulder stability, core strength, and mobility. While holding a kettlebell or dumbbell overhead, slowly move from a lying to a standing position while maintaining control of the weight. The Turkish get-up teaches stability and balance, helping you become more aware of your body's positioning during the press.

4. Triceps Strengthening

While the chest and shoulders dominate the bench press, the triceps play a key role in locking out the weight at the top of the lift. Weak triceps can limit your ability to complete the lift, especially when pressing heavy loads.

- **Triceps Dips**: Triceps dips are a great accessory movement for building triceps strength. Use parallel bars or a bench to perform the dips, lowering yourself until your upper arms are parallel to the ground. Push back up, focusing on squeezing your triceps at the top of the movement. Adding weight with a dip belt can increase the challenge as you progress.
- **Close-Grip Bench Press**: The close-grip bench press is a variation of the traditional bench press that places greater emphasis on the triceps. By bringing your hands closer together on the bar, you shift more of the workload from the chest to the triceps, helping to build pressing power.
- **Overhead Triceps Extension**: Using a dumbbell or resistance band, perform overhead triceps extensions to target the long head of the triceps. This exercise helps to improve lockout strength during the bench press, particularly during the final phase of the lift.
- **Skull Crushers (Lying Triceps Extensions)**: Lying on a bench, hold a barbell or dumbbells with your arms extended above you. Lower the weights toward your forehead by bending your elbows, and then press them back up. This exercise isolates the triceps and enhances lockout strength, making it an excellent accessory for improving the bench press.

5. Pec and Shoulder Activation

Before you attempt a heavy set of bench presses, it's important to activate the chest and shoulder muscles to ensure optimal performance and reduce the risk of injury. The following exercises can help prime these muscle groups for the lift:

- **Chest Flyes**: Using dumbbells or a cable machine, perform chest flyes to activate the pecs and prepare them for pressing. The wide range of motion in this exercise helps warm up the muscles and improves their activation during the bench press.
- **Incline Dumbbell Presses**: The incline dumbbell press targets the upper chest and shoulders, complementing the flat bench press. By strengthening the upper part of the chest, you create a more balanced pressing motion, leading to improved overall performance.
- **Band Push-Ups**: Adding a resistance band to push-ups increases the difficulty and activates the chest, shoulders, and triceps in a way that mirrors the bench press. The added resistance forces your muscles to work harder, improving endurance and strength for the bench press.

Conclusion

Accessory movements for the bench press are a crucial component of any strength training program. By incorporating exercises that target the rotator cuff, improve shoulder mobility, strengthen stabilizing muscles, and enhance triceps power, you can improve your bench press performance while reducing the risk of injury. Consistent work on these accessory exercises will help you unlock new levels of strength and build a more balanced, resilient upper body. As you progress in your training, these exercises will not only support your bench press but will also contribute to your overall functional strength and performance.

Chapter 9: Overcoming Plateaus in the Bench Press

As you progress in your strength training journey, it's inevitable that you will encounter periods where your bench press progress stalls. These plateaus can be frustrating, but they are a natural part of the training process. Overcoming plateaus is an essential skill for every lifter, and with the right strategies, you can push through them and continue to see gains. In this chapter, we will explore how to identify plateaus, adjust your training program, utilize periodization and tempo variations, and employ mental strategies to break through your limits.

1. Identifying Strength Plateaus

Before diving into solutions, it's important to first understand what constitutes a plateau and how to recognize when you're stuck. A plateau occurs when your performance in a specific lift—like the bench press—stagnates, despite consistent effort and progressive overload. Key indicators of a plateau include:

- **Failure to Increase Weights**: If you've been consistently trying to add weight to the bar but can no longer achieve even small increments, you may have hit a plateau.
- **Diminishing Reps**: If your reps or sets are dropping off or you're unable to maintain previous volume at the same weight, it could be a sign that your body is no longer adapting to the training stimulus.
- **Feeling Stagnant**: A lack of motivation, persistent fatigue, or feelings of frustration can indicate that you're no longer experiencing the same level of progress. Training becomes more mentally taxing, and recovery takes longer.

Identifying a plateau early on allows you to take corrective action before it severely hampers your long-term progress.

2. Adjusting the Program

The first step to overcoming a plateau is to change your training approach. Constantly doing the same exercises, rep schemes, and intensities can lead to adaptation, where the body no longer responds to the stimulus in a productive way. Here are a few strategies for breaking through that plateau:

- **Change Your Rep Scheme**: The bench press can be trained effectively with a variety of rep schemes, including low reps (1-5) for strength, moderate reps (6-10) for hypertrophy, and higher reps (12-15) for endurance. If you've been stuck in a certain rep range for a while, shifting to a different rep scheme can reignite progress. For example, if you've been working in the 6-10 rep range, try dropping the weight and training in the 1-5 rep range with heavier loads for a few weeks. This can help you build maximal strength and activate different muscle fibers.
- **Increase Volume**: If you're consistently lifting heavy but not getting the volume necessary for growth, you may need to increase the number of sets or reps. Volume overload can stimulate further muscle growth and strength increases. For example, instead of doing 4 sets of 6 reps, increase to 5 or 6 sets of 8-10 reps. The additional volume will push your muscles to adapt and grow.
- **Change the Tempo**: Adjusting the tempo of your bench press reps can increase time under tension (TUT) and challenge your muscles in new ways. Instead of lifting with a standard 2-1-2 tempo (2 seconds up, 1 second pause, 2 seconds down), try a slower tempo, such as 4-1-4, to increase the intensity of the lift. The slower eccentric phase (lowering the bar) helps develop muscle control and may aid in overcoming sticking points during the lift.

- **Deloading**: If you've been pushing hard for several weeks, your body may need a break. Deloading involves reducing the intensity or volume of your workouts for a short period—usually one week—to allow your body to recover and reset. This can help break the cycle of stagnation and prevent overtraining.

3. Periodization

Periodization is a key concept in strength training that involves cycling through different phases of intensity and volume to prevent stagnation and optimize long-term progress. By structuring your training in cycles, you give your body time to recover and adapt, while progressively overloading the muscles. Here are the main types of periodization you can apply to your bench press training:

- **Linear Periodization**: This approach involves gradually increasing the intensity of your training while decreasing the volume. For example, you might start with higher volume (e.g., 4 sets of 8 reps) and progressively increase the load while reducing the reps (e.g., 4 sets of 5 reps, then 3 sets of 3 reps). Linear periodization is effective for beginners and intermediate lifters, as it provides steady and predictable progress.

- **Undulating Periodization**: This method alternates between different rep ranges and intensities on a weekly or even daily basis. For example, you might do a heavy day (1-3 reps), a moderate day (6-8 reps), and a light day (10-12 reps) within the same week. This approach provides variety, reduces monotony, and helps prevent plateaus by continuously challenging the muscles in different ways.

- **Conjugate Periodization**: This method combines strength, speed, and hypertrophy training by using different methods within the same week. For example, you could focus on maximal strength with lower reps and higher weights one day, then work on explosive power or speed with lighter weights and faster reps on another day. Conjugate periodization helps break through plateaus by targeting various aspects of strength and muscle development.

Each of these approaches can be tailored to your specific training goals and experience level, ensuring you keep progressing and breaking through plateaus in your bench press performance.

4. Mental Strategies to Push Past Limits

Overcoming plateaus isn't just about changing your workout routine; your mindset plays a huge role in pushing through tough moments in training. Here are some mental strategies to help you break through mental and physical barriers:

- **Visualization**: Visualization is a powerful technique used by top athletes. Before hitting the bench press, mentally rehearse the movement. Visualize yourself successfully pushing the barbell off your chest with perfect form and power. This helps build confidence and prepares you mentally for a successful lift.
- **Positive Self-Talk**: When you're struggling to progress, it's easy to fall into negative thinking patterns. Reframe your inner dialogue by focusing on your strengths. Tell yourself, "I am strong," or "I have the power to push through this." Positive affirmations help cultivate resilience and can make a big difference when attempting heavy lifts.
- **Set Mini Goals**: Instead of focusing solely on the end goal, set smaller, incremental targets along the way. For example, aim to add 2.5 kg (5 pounds) to each side of the bar every week, or try to add an extra rep to your sets. Breaking down big goals into smaller, achievable targets will help you stay motivated and make progress over time.
- **Train with a Partner**: Having a lifting partner can help you push past plateaus by offering motivation, encouragement, and assistance. A training partner can help spot you during heavy lifts, give you feedback on your form, and challenge you to push harder than you would on your own.

- **Embrace Failure**: While the idea of failing can be daunting, learning how to handle failure is essential for growth. Training to failure on certain sets or reps can be beneficial for developing mental toughness. It teaches you to push beyond your comfort zone and build resilience.

5. Incorporating Advanced Techniques

If you've been lifting for a while and have mastered the basics, you may need to incorporate more advanced techniques to break through plateaus. Some methods to consider include:

- **Training to Failure**: As previously mentioned, training to failure involves pushing yourself until you can no longer complete a full rep. While this can be physically taxing, it can stimulate muscle growth and break through strength plateaus when used strategically.

- **Accommodating Resistance**: Adding resistance bands or chains to your bench press is an effective way to increase resistance at the top of the movement, where you're the strongest. This helps increase power output and improves lockout strength. It's especially useful for athletes looking to develop maximal strength in their presses.

- **Board Presses and Floor Presses**: Both board presses (where a board is placed on the chest to limit range of motion) and floor presses (where you press from the floor to reduce the range of motion) are variations that target the lockout phase of the lift, where many lifters struggle. These variations help build triceps strength and break through plateaus.

Conclusion

Plateaus in the bench press are a natural part of any lifter's journey, but they don't have to be permanent. By recognizing the signs of a plateau early, adjusting your program with strategies like periodization, varying your training volume, tempo, and rep schemes, and utilizing mental tricks to push past limits, you can overcome these obstacles and continue to progress. Remember, strength building is a marathon, not a sprint. Embrace the challenge, stay consistent, and trust in your ability to break through every plateau.

Chapter 10: Advanced Bench Press Techniques

After mastering the fundamentals of the bench press, reaching the next level in strength training requires incorporating advanced techniques. These techniques go beyond the basics of form, reps, and weight and are designed to help you push past your current limitations, build even more strength, and enhance your pressing power. Whether you are a seasoned lifter or someone looking to break through a plateau, these advanced strategies can maximize your bench press potential.

In this chapter, we will explore some of the most effective advanced bench press techniques, including training to failure, accommodating resistance using bands and chains, and various bench press variations like board presses and floor presses. With the right application, these techniques will add both strength and variety to your workout regimen, leading to greater long-term progress.

1. Training to Failure and Beyond

One of the most powerful methods for increasing strength and muscle hypertrophy is training to failure. This technique involves performing an exercise until you cannot complete another rep with good form. Training to failure recruits more muscle fibers, promotes greater muscle growth, and enhances the strength adaptations needed to break plateaus.

Why Training to Failure Works:

- **Maximal Effort:** Pushing your muscles to their absolute limit activates all muscle fibers, particularly the fast-twitch fibers, which are responsible for explosive strength.
- **Increased Time Under Tension:** Reaching failure extends the time your muscles are under tension, which is a critical factor for muscle growth.
- **Mental Toughness:** Training to failure builds mental fortitude, helping you push through discomfort and fatigue, which is essential for long-term progress.

How to Use Training to Failure:

- **Use sparingly:** While effective, training to failure can be taxing on the body and increase the risk of overtraining if used excessively. It's best to apply this technique in cycles, such as once every 2-4 weeks.
- **Progressive Overload:** Start with a weight you can safely press for 8-10 reps. As you progress, push yourself to failure with that weight, striving to increase the number of reps over time. Eventually, increase the load once you consistently hit failure with your current weight.

Key Considerations:

- **Spotter:** Always train to failure with a spotter, especially when attempting heavy weights, to ensure your safety.
- **Form and Control:** Even when pushing to failure, maintaining proper form is critical. Do not sacrifice form for extra reps, as this can lead to injury.

2. Accommodating Resistance: Bands and Chains

Accommodating resistance is a method used to increase the load during different phases of the lift. Unlike traditional lifting, where the resistance is constant throughout the movement, accommodating resistance (using bands or chains) changes the load depending on the position of the lift. This allows you to apply more resistance during the stronger portion of the lift (near lockout) and less resistance during the weaker portion (the bottom of the press).

Using Bands: Bands are typically attached to the barbell and anchored to the floor or the rack. As you press the bar upward, the bands stretch and increase the resistance. This is especially beneficial for improving the lockout portion of the bench press.

Using Chains: Chains work similarly to bands but provide a different feel. As you lift the barbell, more chains come off the ground, adding incremental weight to the lift. Chains are often used for strength-focused training, particularly in the lockout phase, and can be more forgiving than bands in terms of consistency.

Benefits of Accommodating Resistance:

- **Overcoming Sticking Points:** Bands and chains are particularly effective for strengthening weak points in your lift, especially when you struggle with the top portion of the bench press (the lockout).
- **Increased Power Output:** The gradual increase in resistance during the pressing phase helps improve power and speed, particularly beneficial for athletic performance and explosive strength.
- **Variety:** Adding bands or chains introduces variability to your training, preventing your body from adapting to the same stimulus over time.

How to Implement:

- **Start Slowly:** If you've never used bands or chains before, start with lighter resistance to get a feel for the change in loading. Gradually increase the resistance over time as you build strength and confidence.
- **Alternate With Conventional Training:** Use bands or chains in one of your weekly bench press sessions, while continuing your normal bench press program during other workouts to prevent overtraining.

3. Board Presses: Targeting the Lockout

Board presses are an excellent way to focus on the lockout phase of the bench press—the portion of the lift where many lifters fail. By using a board placed on your chest (or just above it), you reduce the range of motion and eliminate the need to press the bar through the entire movement, isolating the top portion of the press.

Why Board Presses Work:

- **Strengthens Lockout:** The lockout phase often requires maximal triceps and shoulder activation. Board presses help target and strengthen these muscle groups by removing the initial stretch reflex that occurs when the bar touches the chest.
- **Improves Confidence:** For those who struggle with the top portion of the bench press, board presses allow you to use heavier weights, boosting confidence when attempting a full bench press.

How to Do a Board Press:

- **Choose the Right Board Height:** Typically, boards come in different heights (2, 3, or 4 inches), and you can experiment with different heights depending on where you struggle most in the lift. A 2-inch board is ideal for targeting the mid-range, while a 3 or 4-inch board focuses on the lockout.
- **Set Up the Board:** Have a spotter place the board on your chest before you press. Lower the bar to the board, pause for a moment, and then press the bar back up.
- **Focus on Form:** Even though you're using a partial range of motion, maintain the same pressing mechanics as you would in a full bench press. Keep your back tight, elbows tucked, and focus on explosive force.

When to Use Board Presses:

- **Strength Focus:** Use board presses when you are looking to increase lockout strength or break through plateaus in the upper portion of the lift.
- **Periodization:** Incorporate them into a strength phase, such as after a few weeks of regular bench press training, to give your muscles a new challenge and increase triceps power.

4. Floor Presses: Engaging the Triceps and Shoulders

Floor presses are another variation that reduces the range of motion but places greater emphasis on the triceps and shoulders. Instead of performing the press from a bench, you lie flat on the floor, limiting the movement to the upper portion of the press.

Why Floor Presses Work:

- **Reduced Elbow Stress:** For individuals with shoulder issues or those looking to reduce strain on the elbows, floor presses can be a great option. The limited range of motion prevents overstretching and promotes shoulder health.
- **Triceps Activation:** With the bar starting from a lower position, the floor press emphasizes tricep strength in a way that regular bench pressing doesn't. This is ideal for improving overall pressing power and performance.

How to Perform the Floor Press:

- **Setup:** Lie on the floor and set the barbell up on the pins of a squat rack or have a spotter hand it to you. Your feet will remain flat on the floor, and your back should stay neutral, just as with a standard bench press.
- **Lower the Bar:** Slowly lower the bar until your upper arms are flat on the floor, keeping the elbows tucked. Ensure that your elbows don't flare out too much, as this could cause shoulder strain.
- **Press Back Up:** Press the bar upward with control, focusing on squeezing your triceps and chest as you reach the top. Engage your core throughout the movement.

When to Use Floor Presses:

- **Triceps Focus:** Use floor presses when you want to specifically target the triceps and shoulders. It is especially beneficial if you've reached a plateau in the top portion of the lift and need to strengthen the triceps for better lockout power.
- **Strength Cycles:** Incorporate them in cycles where your goal is maximal strength, particularly after several weeks of full-range bench pressing.

Conclusion

Mastering the bench press involves more than just learning the proper form and progressively adding weight. Advanced techniques like training to failure, using accommodating resistance, and incorporating variations like board and floor presses are essential for breaking through plateaus and continuing to build strength. By strategically integrating these techniques into your training program, you can target weak points, enhance power output, and push past the limits that previously held you back.

With consistent effort, focus, and smart application of these advanced strategies, you can elevate your bench press performance and take your strength to new heights.

Chapter 11: The Military Press: Overview and Benefits

The military press is a fundamental exercise that has long been associated with upper body strength and athletic performance. As one of the most effective movements for developing the shoulders, triceps, and upper chest, the military press is a staple in strength training programs worldwide. In this chapter, we'll delve into the anatomy of the military press, its key benefits, and how it contributes to overall strength development and functional fitness.

1. Anatomy of the Military Press

The military press primarily targets the **deltoid muscles**, which are located on the shoulders. The deltoids consist of three distinct parts:

- **Anterior Deltoid** (front): This part of the shoulder is heavily involved in pressing movements, especially when the arms are raised in front of the body.
- **Lateral Deltoid** (middle): The middle deltoid plays a crucial role in shoulder abduction (moving the arm away from the body) and stabilizing the shoulder during pressing movements.
- **Posterior Deltoid** (rear): Although less engaged in pressing movements, the posterior deltoid provides essential stability and balance to the shoulder joint during overhead presses.

In addition to the deltoids, the military press also works several other muscles:

- **Triceps**: The triceps are responsible for extending the elbow as you push the weight overhead.
- **Upper Chest (Pectoralis Major)**: Though not the primary muscle involved, the upper chest helps stabilize the barbell during the press and is particularly activated when the press is performed with a slight incline or a close grip.
- **Upper Back (Traps, Rhomboids, and Lats)**: These muscles help stabilize the shoulder girdle and assist in preventing excessive shoulder movement during the lift.
- **Core Muscles**: The military press requires a stable core for optimal performance. The abdominals, obliques, and lower back muscles are heavily engaged to provide balance and prevent excessive arching of the lower back.

2. Key Benefits of the Military Press

The military press offers a host of benefits that make it one of the best exercises for developing functional strength and enhancing athletic performance. Below are the key advantages of mastering this lift:

- **Shoulder Strength and Development**: The primary benefit of the military press is the development of shoulder strength and muscle mass. As a compound movement, it recruits multiple muscles and encourages balanced growth of the deltoids, particularly the anterior and lateral heads. Over time, the military press can significantly increase shoulder size and strength.
- **Upper Body Power**: In addition to building shoulder strength, the military press helps develop upper body power. The ability to press heavy weights overhead translates to improved performance in various athletic activities, including throwing, pushing, and lifting movements.
- **Functional Strength**: Unlike machine-based exercises, the military press mimics real-world movements such as lifting heavy objects overhead or pushing against resistance. This functional strength is crucial for daily activities and sports performance, making the military press essential for athletes and anyone seeking to improve their physical capabilities.
- **Core Stability**: The military press engages the core muscles, especially the obliques, rectus abdominis, and erector spinae. This creates a stable platform for pressing and helps improve overall posture and spinal alignment, reducing the risk of injury during other movements.

- **Increased Testosterone Production**: Compound lifts like the military press have been shown to increase testosterone levels, which is beneficial for muscle growth, fat loss, and overall performance. The military press, being a heavy, multi-joint lift, stimulates large amounts of muscle mass, leading to a greater release of anabolic hormones.
- **Improved Overhead Mobility**: Regular practice of the military press increases shoulder mobility and stability, which can improve performance in other lifts, such as the bench press and pull-up. It can also reduce the risk of shoulder injuries by strengthening the rotator cuff and increasing shoulder joint stability.

3. Military Press and Athletic Performance

The military press isn't just about building muscle; it has real-world applications in improving overall athletic performance. The lift contributes to the following areas:

- **Overhead Strength**: Whether it's throwing a football, lifting a barbell in Olympic weightlifting, or performing military-style tasks, overhead strength is essential. The military press improves your ability to generate power in overhead movements, enhancing performance in sports like basketball, volleyball, and swimming.
- **Postural Control**: Because of its emphasis on shoulder stability and core engagement, the military press helps athletes maintain good posture, which is essential for all sports. Proper posture improves breathing, balance, and the ability to produce force, all of which contribute to better athletic performance.
- **Injury Prevention**: The military press strengthens the shoulder and upper back muscles, which are vital for stabilizing the shoulder joint during explosive movements. By building strength and endurance in these muscles, you can protect the shoulders from common injuries, such as rotator cuff strains or shoulder impingements, which are common in sports like swimming and tennis.
- **Cross-Training Benefits**: The military press also complements other lifts such as the bench press, deadlift, and squat. By balancing pushing and pulling movements in your training, you can develop well-rounded strength, improving your overall power, posture, and coordination.

4. Mental Benefits of the Military Press

The military press is not only a physical challenge but also a mental one. Overcoming the psychological hurdles of pressing a heavy barbell overhead requires focus, determination, and discipline. Here are a few mental benefits associated with the military press:

- **Focus and Determination**: The military press demands total concentration, as you must maintain a strong, stable base while pressing the barbell overhead. With each lift, you train your mind to focus and push through discomfort, which translates into improved mental toughness in other areas of life.
- **Confidence Building**: Mastering the military press, especially when progressing to heavier weights, can be an empowering experience. The act of lifting substantial loads overhead builds confidence, not only in the gym but also in daily life. The mental toughness gained from overcoming a challenging lift can boost self-esteem and resilience.
- **Overcoming Limits**: As with other heavy compound lifts, the military press provides an opportunity to push past perceived limits. Each successful lift, whether it's hitting a new personal best or completing a challenging set, reinforces the idea that you are capable of more than you initially thought.

5. Integrating the Military Press into Your Program

While the military press is often considered a specialized lift, it should be a core component of any comprehensive strength training program. Whether your goal is to increase upper body power, improve athletic performance, or enhance overall strength, the military press provides numerous benefits that complement other exercises like the bench press and bent-over rows.

To maximize the effectiveness of the military press in your program:

- **Combine with Other Compound Lifts**: Integrate the military press with other fundamental lifts like the squat, deadlift, and bench press to create a balanced routine. The military press can be done on upper-body focused days, either at the start of the workout for strength development or after other pressing movements for accessory work.
- **Frequency**: For maximum strength gains, aim to train the military press at least once or twice a week, depending on your level of experience and recovery. This frequency allows you to build consistent progress without overtraining.
- **Progressive Overload**: As with any strength exercise, progressive overload is key. Gradually increase the weight, volume, or intensity of your military press over time to ensure continuous improvement. This will stimulate muscle growth and increase overall pressing strength.

Conclusion

The military press is a cornerstone movement in strength training that offers a wide range of physical, functional, and mental benefits. It develops the shoulders, enhances upper body power, and improves overall athleticism. Whether you are an athlete, a bodybuilder, or someone looking to increase general strength and functionality, incorporating the military press into your training routine is essential. By mastering this lift, you'll build a strong foundation for total body strength, improve athletic performance, and develop the mental fortitude to push past your limits.

Chapter 12: Perfecting Your Form

The military press is one of the most effective upper body exercises for building strength, power, and shoulder stability. However, mastering the technique is essential not only for maximizing performance but also for preventing injury. In this chapter, we will break down the perfect form for the military press, focusing on the key elements of posture, core engagement, and pressing strategy to ensure you are pressing safely and effectively.

1. Setting Up for Success

A strong military press begins with a solid setup. Ensuring your body is positioned correctly from the start will lay the foundation for a safe and efficient lift.

- **Foot Position**: Start by standing with your feet shoulder-width apart, firmly planted on the floor. Your toes should be pointing straight ahead or slightly outward. This stable base allows you to engage your legs and core during the lift, contributing to better overall power and stability. Keep your feet flat, pressing them into the floor to maintain balance throughout the movement.
- **Grip**: The grip should be just outside shoulder width. When gripping the bar, your wrists should be straight—not bent back—so that the bar rests comfortably in your palms. A false grip (thumbs around the bar) or a regular grip (thumbs wrapped around) can both work, but ensure that your wrists remain aligned and stable throughout the lift.
- **Bar Placement**: The bar should rest just above your clavicles when starting the lift. This position ensures that the bar is in the most efficient place to press upward without excessive strain on the shoulders. If the bar is too high on your chest or too low, you'll struggle to press effectively.
- **Engaging Your Core**: Before you begin the press, take a deep breath and brace your core. This is crucial for maintaining stability during the lift. Imagine trying to push your belly button into your spine as you tighten your abdominals and lower back muscles. A strong core prevents excessive arching in the lower back and ensures that the force you generate from your legs and torso is transferred efficiently through your arms.

- **Scapular Retraction**: Pull your shoulder blades back and down (as if trying to pinch a pencil between them). This posture helps to stabilize the shoulder joint and reduces the risk of shoulder impingement or strain during the press. Keeping your shoulders retracted will also allow for a stronger, more controlled movement.

2. The Pressing Movement

Now that you're set up with the right position, let's break down the pressing motion itself. Mastering the technique is key to both lifting heavier and maintaining long-term joint health.

- **Initiate with the Legs**: Although the military press is an upper-body movement, the legs play a significant role in stabilizing your body during the lift. Before you begin the press, engage your glutes and quads by pushing your feet into the floor. This helps lock your body into place and prepares you for a strong lift.

- **Pressing the Bar**: Begin by pressing the barbell directly overhead in a straight line. The bar should follow a vertical path, not drifting forward or backward. As you press, your elbows should move from a slightly forward position to fully locked out above the shoulders. Avoid flaring your elbows too much, as this can place unnecessary strain on the shoulders.

- **Head and Neck Position**: As you press the bar up, it's important to slightly move your head back to allow the bar to pass directly over your face. Once the bar is past your forehead, your head should return to a neutral position. Keeping your head aligned with your spine helps maintain a strong base of support while preventing unnecessary tension in the neck.

- **Full Extension**: At the top of the press, your arms should be fully extended with your elbows locked out. At this point, your shoulders, elbows, and wrists should form a straight line. The bar should be stacked directly over your body to maintain the best mechanical advantage. Avoid leaning back or excessively arching your back at the top of the press. Keeping a neutral spine is crucial for minimizing the risk of injury.

3. The Descent and Reset

After reaching the top of the press, you must carefully control the bar as you lower it. While it may be tempting to let the bar drop, maintaining control over the descent is vital for both safety and muscle engagement.

- **Controlled Descent**: Lower the bar slowly and with control, keeping the same path as when pressing upward. Resist the urge to let gravity take over. A slow, controlled descent increases time under tension and provides an additional strength-building benefit. Aim for about a 3-4 second lowering phase to maximize muscle engagement in the shoulders and triceps.
- **Breathing**: As you lower the bar, exhale slowly and ensure you are maintaining tension in your core. You can take another deep breath at the bottom of the movement to brace yourself before initiating the next rep. Keep a consistent breathing pattern throughout the lift to maintain stability and power.
- **Repetitions and Pauses**: For optimal strength gains, it's important to decide whether you want to train for maximal strength or hypertrophy. If your goal is strength, consider performing each rep with minimal rest at the bottom and focusing on quick, explosive movements. If your goal is hypertrophy or endurance, you may want to incorporate a brief pause at the bottom of each rep, ensuring your muscles are under constant tension for a longer period.

4. Common Mistakes to Avoid

While the military press is a relatively simple movement, several common mistakes can hinder progress and increase the risk of injury. Here are a few to watch out for:

- **Arching the Lower Back**: One of the most common mistakes in the military press is over-arching the lower back to generate more power. This can cause strain on the spine and lead to long-term injury. Ensure that your core is engaged and that your lower back stays neutral throughout the movement.
- **Flaring the Elbows**: Letting your elbows flare out excessively during the press places undue stress on the shoulder joints. Keep your elbows close to your body and avoid excessive outward motion.
- **Not Using Full Range of Motion**: A common mistake is not lowering the bar to the chest or not fully extending the arms at the top of the movement. Both of these limit the potential for muscle growth and strength development. Be sure to use the full range of motion to activate all the muscle groups involved.
- **Allowing the Bar to Drift**: The bar should stay in a straight line overhead. Allowing the bar to drift forward or backward can negatively affect your shoulder health and decrease the effectiveness of the movement. Focus on keeping the bar over your body.

5. Pressing Strategies for Shoulder Health

The military press is an incredible exercise for building upper body strength, but it can also put significant strain on the shoulders if not executed properly. Here are some strategies to ensure shoulder health as you press:

- **Warm-Up Properly**: Before attempting heavy military press sets, it's essential to warm up the shoulder joint and surrounding muscles. Use dynamic stretches and mobility exercises, such as arm circles, shoulder dislocations with a resistance band, and light dumbbell presses to increase blood flow to the area and prepare for the heavy work ahead.
- **Shoulder Mobility**: A lack of shoulder mobility can limit your range of motion and lead to poor pressing technique. Incorporating mobility drills into your warm-up routine, such as external rotations, wall slides, and chest openers, can help improve your flexibility and range of motion for pressing exercises.
- **Rotator Cuff Health**: Regularly performing rotator cuff exercises can help strengthen the muscles that stabilize the shoulder joint. Movements like internal and external rotations with a resistance band or light dumbbells can help keep the rotator cuff healthy and reduce the risk of injury.
- **Overhead Press Variations**: While the military press is fantastic for building shoulder strength, incorporating other overhead pressing movements, such as dumbbell presses or incline presses, can help target different parts of the shoulder and reduce the risk of overuse injuries.

6. Conclusion

Mastering the military press is essential for building upper body strength, power, and functional movement. By focusing on proper setup, posture, and pressing technique, you can maximize your performance and reduce the risk of injury. Remember to engage your core, maintain a neutral spine, and keep the bar path straight to ensure an effective and safe press. With consistent practice and attention to form, you'll develop stronger, more resilient shoulders that will serve as a foundation for all your lifting endeavors.

Chapter 13: Accessory Movements for the Military Press

While the military press is a powerful exercise on its own, incorporating accessory movements into your routine can significantly enhance your shoulder strength, stability, and mobility. These supplementary exercises target the smaller muscle groups involved in pressing, improving your overall performance and helping to prevent injuries. In this chapter, we'll explore key accessory movements that will complement and strengthen your military press, focusing on rotator cuff exercises, scapular stability, triceps and deltoid strengthening, and essential shoulder mobility drills.

1. Rotator Cuff Exercises

The rotator cuff is a group of four small muscles that stabilize the shoulder joint, playing a critical role in preventing injury during pressing movements. Weakness or imbalances in these muscles can lead to shoulder pain, poor posture, and reduced pressing power. Strengthening the rotator cuff should be a priority for anyone who regularly performs the military press.

External Rotations

- *How to do it:* Attach a resistance band to a sturdy object at elbow height. Stand with your side to the attachment point and hold the band with your outside hand. Keep your elbow at a 90-degree angle and press your shoulder back. Rotate your arm outward, keeping your elbow pinned to your side, until your forearm is parallel to the ground. Return to the starting position with control.
- *Reps:* 3 sets of 10–12 reps per side.

Internal Rotations

- *How to do it:* Stand with your body facing the resistance band or cable attachment. Grasp the handle with the hand nearest to the attachment point. Keeping your elbow at 90 degrees, rotate your arm inward until your forearm is across your body. Slowly return to the starting position.
- *Reps:* 3 sets of 10–12 reps per side.

Prone Reverse Flyes

- *How to do it:* Lie face down on a bench, holding light dumbbells in each hand. With your arms extended straight below you, lift the dumbbells out to your sides, squeezing your shoulder blades together at the top. Lower back to the start position with control.
- *Reps:* 3 sets of 12–15 reps.

2. Scapular Stability Exercises

The scapula plays a vital role in overhead pressing, and poor scapular stability can limit your ability to press effectively. Strengthening the muscles around the scapula, such as the rhomboids, traps, and serratus anterior, will improve your pressing mechanics and help protect your shoulders.

Scapular Push-Ups

- *How to do it*: Start in a push-up position, with your hands directly under your shoulders. Without bending your elbows, squeeze your shoulder blades together, lowering your body slightly. Then, push your shoulder blades apart, raising your torso. This movement should come from your shoulder blades, not your arms.
- *Reps*: 3 sets of 12-15 reps.

Face Pulls

- *How to do it*: Set a rope attachment on a cable machine at face height. Grab the rope with both hands, and step back with your arms extended in front of you. Pull the rope towards your face, keeping your elbows high and wide. Focus on squeezing your shoulder blades together at the peak of the movement.
- *Reps*: 3 sets of 10-12 reps.

Wall Slides

- *How to do it*: Stand with your back against a wall, with your feet about 6 inches away. Press your lower back, upper back, and head into the wall. Place your arms in a "W" position, with elbows bent and forearms against the wall. Slowly slide your arms up the wall, maintaining contact between your arms and the wall. Lower back down with control.
- *Reps*: 3 sets of 8-10 reps.

3. Strengthening the Triceps

The triceps are responsible for locking out the military press at the top of the movement. Strong triceps not only help you push the barbell overhead but also reduce fatigue during high-rep pressing. Incorporating triceps-focused accessory exercises will help improve pressing endurance and strength.

Triceps Dips

- *How to do it:* Using parallel bars, support your body with your arms fully extended. Lower your body by bending your elbows to about 90 degrees, keeping your chest up and your body vertical. Push back up to the starting position.
- *Reps:* 3 sets of 8–12 reps.

Close-Grip Bench Press

- *How to do it:* Set up on the bench press as you normally would, but with your hands positioned about shoulder-width apart or slightly narrower. Lower the bar to your chest, keeping your elbows close to your body, then press back up.
- *Reps:* 3 sets of 5–8 reps.

Overhead Triceps Extension

- *How to do it*: Hold a dumbbell or a barbell overhead with both hands. Lower the weight behind your head by bending your elbows, keeping your upper arms close to your head. Press the weight back up to the starting position.
- *Reps*: 3 sets of 10-12 reps.

4. Deltoid Strengthening

Strong deltoids are essential for a powerful military press, as they bear the brunt of the load during the movement. Targeting all three heads of the deltoids—the anterior (front), lateral (middle), and posterior (rear)—will enhance your overall pressing strength and shoulder stability.

Lateral Raises

- *How to do it*: Stand with a dumbbell in each hand at your sides. With a slight bend in your elbows, raise your arms out to the sides until they are parallel to the ground. Lower back to the starting position with control.
- *Reps*: 3 sets of 12-15 reps.

Front Raises

- *How to do it*: Hold a dumbbell in each hand in front of your thighs. With a slight bend in the elbows, raise the dumbbells in front of you until your arms are parallel to the ground. Lower back to the starting position slowly.
- *Reps*: 3 sets of 10-12 reps.

Arnold Press

- *How to do it*: Hold a dumbbell in each hand in front of your shoulders, palms facing your body. As you press the dumbbells overhead, rotate your wrists so your palms face forward at the top of the movement. Reverse the motion as you lower the dumbbells back down.
- *Reps*: 3 sets of 8-10 reps.

5. Shoulder Mobility Drills

Maintaining adequate shoulder mobility is crucial for pressing exercises, especially the military press. Limited shoulder mobility can prevent you from achieving a proper range of motion and increase the risk of injury. Incorporating mobility drills into your routine will enhance your pressing performance and shoulder health.

Band Pull-Aparts

- *How to do it*: Hold a resistance band with both hands in front of you at shoulder height. Keep your arms straight and pull the band apart, squeezing your shoulder blades together. Slowly return to the starting position.
- *Reps*: 3 sets of 15–20 reps.

Shoulder Dislocations

- *How to do it*: Hold a resistance band or PVC pipe with a wide grip in front of your body. Slowly raise the band or pipe overhead, keeping your arms straight. Continue the movement behind your body, stretching your shoulders and chest. Reverse the motion to return to the starting position.
- *Reps*: 3 sets of 10–12 reps.

6. Conclusion

Incorporating accessory movements for the military press is essential for improving shoulder strength, stability, and mobility. By targeting the rotator cuff, enhancing scapular stability, strengthening the triceps and deltoids, and focusing on shoulder mobility, you'll build a more resilient and powerful pressing foundation. These exercises will help you overcome plateaus, prevent injury, and ultimately enhance your performance in the military press.

Chapter 14: Overcoming Plateaus in the Military Press

No matter how consistent and dedicated you are, it's inevitable: you'll hit a plateau at some point in your strength journey. The military press, with its demand on shoulder stability, triceps strength, and core engagement, can present unique challenges when progress seems to stall. This chapter will explore strategies to break through plateaus in the military press by utilizing deload phases, adjusting rep schemes, focusing on recovery, and targeting weak points in your lift.

1. Understanding Plateaus

A plateau occurs when you stop making progress despite continued effort. In the context of the military press, this may manifest as being unable to increase the weight lifted, or even feeling like your strength has regressed. There are several reasons plateaus happen, including:

- **Adaptation**: Your body has adapted to your current training routine, and your muscles no longer respond to the same stimuli.
- **Overtraining**: Insufficient rest, too much volume, or not enough recovery between sessions can cause fatigue to accumulate, leading to stagnation.
- **Weak Links**: A particular muscle or movement pattern may be limiting your ability to press heavier weights, such as weak triceps or poor scapular stability.

Breaking through these plateaus requires a combination of training modifications, recovery strategies, and mental toughness.

2. Deload Strategies

One of the most effective tools for overcoming a plateau is incorporating deload weeks into your training program. Deloading is a planned reduction in volume or intensity, allowing your body time to recover from accumulated stress and rebuild muscle fibers stronger. It's crucial to give your muscles a break to ensure long-term progress.

When to Deload

- Persistent soreness or joint pain
- A sudden decrease in performance
- Mental burnout or lack of motivation

How to Deload

- **Reducing Weight**: Lower the load to about 50-60% of your 1RM (one-rep max) and focus on maintaining form rather than pushing for new personal records.
- **Cutting Volume**: Reduce the number of sets or reps per exercise.
- **Lowering Frequency**: Instead of training the military press twice a week, reduce it to once, or incorporate lighter accessory exercises to maintain movement patterns without taxing the shoulders excessively.

Deloading allows the body to replenish energy stores, repair muscle fibers, and reset for future growth.

3. Adjusting Rep Schemes

Changing up your rep scheme can help shock your muscles into new growth, sparking further progress. If you've been following a standard 4x6 approach for a while, switching up your rep range can provide a fresh stimulus.

Low-Rep, High-Weight Training

Example

Higher-Rep, Moderate-Weight Training

Example

- **Pyramid Sets**: Gradually increasing weight while decreasing reps (e.g., 10 reps at 50%, 8 reps at 60%, 6 reps at 70%) can allow you to progressively overload while targeting different energy systems and muscle fibers.
- **Wave Loading**: In wave loading, you alternate between heavy, moderate, and light sets within a training cycle. For example, on one day, you may work in the 1-3 rep range, followed by a week with 4-6 reps, and then a light week with 8-10 reps. This variety will stimulate different muscle fibers and help overcome a plateau.

4. The Importance of Rest and Recovery

Rest and recovery are often overlooked but are crucial in overcoming plateaus. If you're constantly pushing hard without adequate recovery, your body won't have the chance to repair and grow stronger. Recovery plays a pivotal role in muscle adaptation, and neglecting it could be the main reason for your stagnation.

- **Sleep**: Ensure you're getting at least 7-9 hours of quality sleep per night. Sleep is when muscle repair and growth occur, and poor sleep quality can directly impair your performance in the gym.
- **Active Recovery**: Incorporating lighter activities like stretching, foam rolling, and mobility drills into your weekly routine will keep blood flowing to your muscles and improve joint health. Active recovery reduces muscle tightness and prevents overuse injuries.
- **Nutrition**: Adequate protein intake (roughly 1.6-2.2 grams per kilogram of body weight) is essential to support muscle recovery and repair. Ensure you're also getting enough carbohydrates to replenish glycogen stores and fats for hormonal health. A recovery meal post-workout that includes protein and carbs can help kickstart the repair process.

5. Variations to Target Weak Points in the Lift

Sometimes, the issue lies with specific weaknesses that hinder your press. Targeting these weak points with accessory movements can help improve your military press performance.

- **Triceps Strengthening**: If you struggle to lock out at the top of your press, your triceps may need more focus. Incorporate exercises like close-grip bench presses, dips, skull crushers, and overhead triceps extensions to build more pressing power.
- **Shoulder Mobility and Stability**: Limited range of motion or poor scapular control could be holding back your press. Incorporate shoulder mobility drills, band pull-aparts, face pulls, and scapular push-ups to enhance shoulder health and prevent compensatory movement patterns.
- **Core Stability**: A weak core can make it difficult to maintain an upright posture during the military press. Strengthen your core with exercises like planks, hanging leg raises, and ab wheel rollouts to maintain proper alignment while pressing overhead.
- **Explosiveness**: If your press lacks speed or you're struggling with heavier weights, incorporating explosive variations can help. Try push presses, where you use leg drive to initiate the lift, or even incorporate some Olympic lifts like the clean and press, which will train your ability to generate power quickly and efficiently.

6. Mental Strategies to Push Through Plateaus

Strength training is as much a mental challenge as it is a physical one. Mental toughness can be the difference between stagnation and progress, especially when facing a plateau.

- **Visualization**: Spend time visualizing your successful military press, from setting up to locking out the bar overhead. Visualizing success can help build confidence and reinforce proper form.
- **Goal Setting**: Break down your long-term goals into short, actionable steps. Focus on small wins, such as adding an extra rep or increasing the weight by 5 pounds. These small successes add up and can help push you through a plateau.
- **Mental Toughness Techniques**: When you feel the weight getting heavy, use mental cues to maintain focus and strength. Phrases like "drive through the floor" or "push the ceiling away" can help reinforce the movement and keep you focused on completing the rep.
- **Tracking Progress**: Keep a training log to track progress, even if the numbers aren't immediately increasing. Reviewing your progress can help you identify patterns, understand your training cycles, and give you the confidence to push through when you hit a wall.

7. Conclusion

Overcoming plateaus in the military press requires a multifaceted approach. By incorporating deload weeks, adjusting rep schemes, focusing on recovery, and targeting weak points, you can break through strength barriers and continue progressing in your training. Remember that plateaus are a natural part of the training process, and with the right adjustments, you'll come out stronger and more resilient. Keep pushing forward, and you'll soon find yourself pressing heavier weights with greater efficiency and control.

Chapter 15: Advanced Military Press Techniques

The military press is one of the foundational lifts for developing upper body strength, and once you've mastered its basic form, you can begin exploring advanced techniques to take your pressing power to the next level. These techniques will focus on maximizing your power, speed, and endurance, all while maintaining healthy shoulder mechanics and preventing injury. Whether you want to increase your 1-rep max or use the military press to enhance athletic performance, these advanced strategies will help you reach your goals.

1. Strict Press vs. Push Press vs. Jerk

While the military press is often referred to as a "strict press," there are variations of the movement that allow for greater weight to be lifted by utilizing the legs and hips. Understanding when and how to incorporate these variations can drastically improve your overall performance.

Strict Press (Overhead Press)

- *When to use it*: Use the strict press for building shoulder strength and stability. It's ideal for focusing on form, keeping the core engaged, and avoiding using momentum.
- *Key tip*: Focus on keeping your core tight and pressing the bar in a straight line. Any movement forward or backward in the bar path can cause you to lose efficiency and power.

Push Press

- *How to perform it:* Start with the barbell at shoulder height, engage your core, and dip slightly by bending your knees and hips. Then, explosively drive through your legs and hips, transferring the energy upwards to help press the bar overhead. Finish by locking your arms out at the top.
- *When to use it:* The push press is ideal for developing explosive power and improving strength endurance. It also helps you lift heavier loads than with a strict press, which can translate to increased muscle mass and strength in the upper body.
- *Key tip:* Focus on keeping the dip shallow—just enough to generate momentum—and ensure the bar travels in a straight line overhead to avoid unnecessary strain on the shoulders.

Jerk

- *How to perform it*: Start with the barbell at shoulder height. Dip down quickly by bending your knees and hips, then drive upward with your legs and aggressively "split" your stance into a front lunge while pressing the bar overhead. Catch the bar in the split position, then stand up to lock out your arms and feet simultaneously.
- *When to use it*: The jerk is perfect for maximizing your overhead lifting potential and improving your power output. It's especially beneficial for athletes who require explosive upper-body power, such as sprinters, football players, or crossfitters.
- *Key tip*: Focus on maintaining an explosive drive with the legs and a smooth transition between the dip and press. Your arms should remain straight during the split, and your catch should be controlled and stable.

2. Power and Speed Emphasis

Incorporating a focus on power and speed into your military press routine can help you break through strength plateaus and develop greater athletic performance. This is especially important for athletes who need to generate maximal force quickly—whether for sprinting, jumping, or combat sports.

Speed Work

- *How to do it*: Use about 50-70% of your 1-rep max and perform each repetition as explosively as possible. Rest only briefly between sets (around 45-60 seconds) to keep the intensity high.
- *When to use it*: Speed work is best utilized as part of a dynamic effort day within your weekly routine. This will increase power output, which is crucial for improving performance in both the press and other athletic movements.
- *Key tip*: Focus on perfecting the form during speed work. Moving the bar explosively with improper form can lead to injury, especially in the shoulders. Ensure the bar follows a straight vertical path to avoid unnecessary strain.

Paused Reps

- *How to do it*: Lower the bar to the chest or just below the chin, and pause for 1-2 seconds before pressing it upward. This eliminates the use of any bounce from the chest, forcing your muscles to initiate the press without relying on momentum.
- *When to use it*: Paused reps are excellent for improving lockout strength and for teaching better control during the press.
- *Key tip*: Keep your core tight and avoid sinking into a "lazy" position during the pause. The emphasis is on staying tight and bracing before pressing the barbell overhead.

3. Using the Military Press for Athletic Training

The military press is not just a strength-building exercise; it can be adapted to enhance performance in sports and other athletic activities. By using specific variations and focusing on the speed and explosiveness of the lift, you can improve functional strength that translates directly to your sport of choice.

Sport-Specific Emphasis

- For **sprinters**, emphasize explosive speed work, using lighter weights and quick, powerful reps to simulate the force needed for a fast start.
- For **football players**, use the push press to increase strength and power, which is essential for tackling, blocking, and pushing through opponents.
- For **athletes in combat sports**, such as MMA or boxing, focus on the strict press to improve shoulder endurance and core stability for throwing punches and clinching.

Olympic Weightlifting Integration

4. Programming Advanced Military Press Techniques

As you incorporate advanced techniques into your military press routine, it's important to properly program these variations to avoid overtraining and ensure continued progress.

- **Periodization**: Incorporating periodization into your training will allow you to cycle between different focuses such as strength, hypertrophy, and power. Plan your programming to include phases of strict pressing, push pressing, and jerking to continually challenge your muscles and avoid stagnation.
- **Combining Lifts**: On days where you focus on strength, emphasize the strict press with heavier weights. On power days, incorporate push presses or speed work with lighter loads. Keep jerk variations reserved for high-explosiveness days or after proper warm-ups to prevent injury.
- **Rest and Recovery**: Advanced lifting techniques can take a toll on the central nervous system (CNS). Ensure adequate rest and recovery between pressing sessions, particularly when incorporating heavy and explosive lifts. This will prevent burnout and support muscle recovery.

5. Conclusion

Mastering the advanced military press techniques—strict press, push press, and jerk—requires a solid foundation of technique and an understanding of how to develop power and speed. By strategically incorporating these variations, emphasizing speed and explosiveness, and adapting the press to fit your sport-specific needs, you'll not only improve your overhead strength but also enhance your overall athletic performance. Whether you're an athlete or a strength enthusiast, these advanced techniques will help you unlock new levels of power and efficiency in your training.

Chapter 16: The Bent-Over Row: Overview and Benefits

The bent-over row is one of the most effective compound exercises for developing the back and enhancing overall upper body strength. While often overshadowed by its pressing counterparts like the bench press and military press, the bent-over row plays a crucial role in achieving a balanced physique and strengthening muscles that are vital for both posture and performance in other lifts. In this chapter, we'll explore the anatomy of the bent-over row, its key benefits, and how it complements pressing exercises to help you build total body strength and improve overall power and performance.

1. Anatomy of the Bent-Over Row

The bent-over row is a horizontal pulling movement that primarily targets the muscles of the back, but it also recruits several other muscle groups. Understanding the anatomy involved will help you appreciate the full benefits of this powerful exercise.

Primary Muscles Targeted

- **Latissimus Dorsi (Lats)**: The largest muscles of the back that give the upper body its characteristic "V" shape. The lats are responsible for shoulder extension and adduction, making them key players in pulling movements.
- **Rhomboids**: Located between the shoulder blades, the rhomboids help retract the scapula and maintain shoulder stability. Strong rhomboids contribute to improved posture and a better ability to perform pressing exercises with proper form.
- **Trapezius (Traps)**: The traps are divided into upper, middle, and lower portions, each responsible for different movements of the scapula and shoulders. The middle traps are heavily engaged during the bent-over row, assisting with scapular retraction and maintaining shoulder integrity.

Secondary Muscles Involved

- **Biceps Brachii**: As with many pulling movements, the biceps play a significant role in the execution of the bent-over row. They are responsible for elbow flexion, helping to draw the weight towards the torso.
- **Rear Deltoids (Posterior Shoulders)**: The posterior deltoids assist in shoulder extension and stabilization during the row. A strong rear deltoid ensures that your shoulders remain stable and healthy during the movement.
- **Erector Spinae**: The muscles along the spine are engaged to stabilize the lower back during the bent-over row. Proper bracing and spinal alignment are crucial to protect the lower back and maintain proper form.

Core Muscles

The core plays a supportive role during the bent-over row by stabilizing the torso and preventing unwanted rotation. Engaging the abdominals, obliques, and lower back muscles helps maintain a strong, rigid position throughout the lift.

2. How Rows Complement Pressing Exercises

The bent-over row works in synergy with pressing exercises like the bench press and military press, ensuring that your training routine develops both the front and back of your body. While pressing movements primarily focus on the chest, shoulders, and triceps, the bent-over row targets the muscles that oppose these pressing motions—primarily the back and biceps.

- **Balancing Pushing and Pulling Movements**: Strengthening the muscles responsible for pulling is vital for maintaining balance in the body. Overemphasis on pressing exercises without corresponding pulling movements can lead to muscle imbalances, poor posture, and increased risk of injury. The bent-over row helps to correct this by promoting a more balanced, functional physique.
- **Improving Pressing Power**: A stronger back translates into more stability during pressing movements. The lats and rhomboids, when properly developed, contribute to shoulder stability and provide a strong base for pressing movements. When you row regularly, you're not only building a bigger back but also improving the ability to press heavier weights overhead or off your chest by providing better scapular stability.
- **Posture and Injury Prevention**: Rows can help counteract the effects of poor posture from prolonged sitting or from performing excessive pressing movements. By strengthening the posterior chain (the back, rear delts, and traps), you enhance your ability to maintain an upright, neutral spine during all lifts, reducing the likelihood of lower back and shoulder injuries.

3. Posture, Strength, and Hypertrophy Benefits

The bent-over row is a powerful exercise for developing strength, muscle mass, and overall athletic performance. Whether you're focused on building muscle or improving your functional strength, the row offers numerous benefits that will complement any training routine.

- **Posture Enhancement**: Modern lifestyles often lead to poor posture, with rounded shoulders and slouched spines becoming common issues. The bent-over row directly targets the muscles responsible for retracting the shoulder blades, which helps correct postural imbalances and promote a more upright stance. Strengthening these muscles encourages proper spinal alignment and reduces the risk of upper back and neck pain.
- **Strength Development**: By consistently incorporating the bent-over row into your routine, you build pulling strength that enhances overall upper body power. This translates to improved performance in other compound lifts, as well as everyday functional movements that require pulling, lifting, or carrying.
- **Hypertrophy (Muscle Growth)**: Rows are an excellent exercise for building muscle mass in the back. They provide an effective stimulus for hypertrophy by targeting multiple muscle groups simultaneously. When performed with proper form and progressively overloaded, the bent-over row can lead to significant gains in back size and density.

Tip for Hypertrophy

4. The Bent-Over Row in a Full-Body Strength Program

Including the bent-over row in your strength training routine helps ensure a well-rounded program that develops both the pushing and pulling muscles. The row complements other compound lifts like the bench press and squat by improving your overall strength, posture, and muscular endurance. Here's how to incorporate rows effectively into your program:

- **Row Frequency**: For optimal back development, include the bent-over row in your routine 1-2 times per week. Depending on your specific goals, you can program rows on upper-body pull days, alongside exercises like deadlifts, pull-ups, or lat pull-downs.
- **Variation**: There are several variations of the bent-over row, each targeting different parts of the back and providing a new stimulus for muscle growth. These include:

- **Barbell Bent-Over Row**: The classic variation that emphasizes overall back development.
- **Dumbbell Rows**: A unilateral exercise that targets each side of the back independently, helping to correct imbalances.
- **T-Bar Rows**: A great variation for building thickness in the mid-back.
- **Pendlay Rows**: A stricter, more explosive version that emphasizes power and strength.

Incorporating Rows with Pressing Exercises

5. Conclusion

The bent-over row is a cornerstone exercise for developing a strong, muscular back, and it complements pressing exercises by improving shoulder stability, posture, and overall upper body strength. Whether you're looking to improve your pressing power, correct postural imbalances, or simply add size to your back, the row is an indispensable part of a well-rounded strength training program. By understanding the anatomy involved, the benefits of the row, and how it complements pressing movements, you'll be better equipped to implement this exercise effectively in your training routine. Keep varying your row variations, focus on perfecting your form, and incorporate progressive overload to continually develop strength and muscle mass.

Chapter 17: Perfecting Your Form: The Bent-Over Row

The bent-over row is one of the most effective exercises for building a strong, powerful back. It's a staple in any serious strength training program, focusing on the development of the latissimus dorsi, traps, rhomboids, and rear deltoids. Mastering the form of the bent-over row is crucial, not just for maximizing muscle development but also for preventing injury and ensuring that you're getting the most out of the movement. In this chapter, we will break down every aspect of the bent-over row, from setup to execution, to help you perfect your form.

1. Setting Up for the Bent-Over Row

Before you even lift the barbell, it's essential to properly set up your body and the equipment. The bent-over row is a compound pulling movement that requires balance and coordination, as well as attention to detail in terms of body mechanics.

Foot Position

Key tip

- **Barbell Setup**: Position the barbell on the floor in front of you. Stand tall with your shins about 1-2 inches away from the bar. Bend down and grip the bar with a pronated (overhand) grip, with your hands roughly shoulder-width apart. Ensure that your grip is firm but relaxed, so you can focus on using your back muscles rather than your arms.
- **Hinge at the Hips**: With a slight bend in your knees, push your hips back (not down) while maintaining a neutral spine. The goal is to lower your torso at a 45-degree angle to the floor. The deeper you hinge, the more you'll engage the lats and rhomboids. A slight bend in the knees will help you maintain balance and allow your hips to travel back without rounding your lower back.

Key tip

Core Engagement

Key tip

2. Proper Back Angle and Posture

Maintaining the right posture throughout the bent-over row is essential to ensure the movement targets the correct muscles and minimizes the risk of injury.

Maintain a Flat Back

Key tip

Retract Your Shoulder Blades

Key tip

3. Grip and Arm Positioning

Your grip and arm positioning during the bent-over row are critical for targeting the correct muscles. While there are different variations of the row (such as underhand or neutral grip), the basic form remains similar across all versions.

Grip Choice

Key tip

Elbow Position

Key tip

4. The Pulling Phase: Breathing and Bracing

As you begin the row, it's important to focus on your breathing and the muscle engagement during the pulling phase. The pulling motion should be powerful but controlled, ensuring that you maintain tension in the target muscles throughout the movement.

Initiate the Pull

Key tip

Breathing

Key tip

Tempo

Key tip

5. Lowering the Bar: Eccentric Phase

The eccentric (lowering) phase of the row is just as important as the concentric (pulling) phase. This is where you can build muscle and strength by controlling the weight as you return to the starting position.

Controlled Descent

Key tip

Reset for Next Rep

6. Common Mistakes and Corrections

As with any exercise, there are common mistakes to avoid when performing the bent-over row. Correcting these mistakes will not only improve your results but also keep you safe from injury.

- **Rounding the Back**: This is the most dangerous mistake you can make when performing the bent-over row. It puts unnecessary strain on the lower back and can lead to serious injury. To fix this, always ensure that your back stays flat and your chest stays up during the lift.
- **Overusing the Arms**: If you rely too much on your arms to complete the row, you won't effectively target your back muscles. Instead, focus on pulling with your elbows and engaging your lats and rhomboids.
- **Jerking the Bar**: Jerking the bar to create momentum reduces the effectiveness of the row and can lead to injury. Always perform the row with controlled, deliberate movements.
- **Elbows Flaring Out**: Flaring your elbows out too much can shift the focus away from the lats and onto the shoulders. To correct this, keep the elbows close to your torso throughout the movement.

7. Conclusion

The bent-over row is a crucial lift for building a strong, muscular back. Mastering the form of the bent-over row ensures that you're getting the most out of the exercise while minimizing the risk of injury. By focusing on your setup, back angle, grip, and breathing, you can perfect the movement and make significant progress in your strength and muscle development. Consistently practicing proper form will help you unlock new levels of performance, whether you're a beginner or an experienced lifter.

Chapter 18: Accessory Movements for Bent-Over Rows

The bent-over row is one of the most effective compound movements for building a strong, balanced back. While the exercise primarily targets the latissimus dorsi (lats), rhomboids, and traps, it also recruits several other muscles that contribute to posture, grip strength, and overall pulling power. However, to maximize the benefits of the bent-over row and prevent muscular imbalances, it is essential to complement it with accessory exercises. These movements help to enhance the muscle groups engaged during the row, address weaknesses, and ensure balanced strength development across the entire body.

In this chapter, we'll explore a variety of accessory movements designed to build pulling power, improve muscle activation, and boost overall performance in the bent-over row. These exercises will strengthen the lats, rhomboids, traps, biceps, forearms, and more, providing a comprehensive approach to developing a well-rounded back and improving your rowing technique.

1. Lat Pulldown

The lat pulldown is an excellent accessory movement to reinforce the muscles used during the bent-over row, particularly the latissimus dorsi. This exercise mimics the pulling motion of a row but in a vertical plane, helping to build a stronger, wider back.

- **How to do it**: Sit at a lat pulldown machine with your knees under the pads. Grip the bar with a wide overhand grip, hands slightly wider than shoulder-width apart. Engage your core and pull the bar down towards your chest, focusing on using your lats rather than your arms. Control the bar as you return it to the starting position.
- **When to use it**: Include lat pulldowns in your accessory routine to develop lat strength and endurance. This movement is particularly useful if you struggle to engage your lats during the bent-over row.
- **Key tip**: Keep your chest proud and your scapula retracted throughout the movement. Avoid swinging or jerking the weight to ensure optimal engagement of the lats.

2. Face Pulls

Face pulls are a great accessory movement for improving the upper back, especially the rear deltoids, traps, and rhomboids. This exercise helps maintain good posture by strengthening the muscles that stabilize the shoulder joint and scapula. Face pulls also improve shoulder mobility and contribute to overall pulling power.

- **How to do it**: Attach a rope handle to a high pulley machine. Grip the rope with both hands, palms facing inward. Step back and pull the rope towards your face, keeping your elbows high and wide, and squeeze your shoulder blades together at the top. Slowly release the rope to the starting position with control.
- **When to use it**: Face pulls should be performed as part of your accessory routine to strengthen the upper back and improve posture. This movement complements the horizontal pulling of the bent-over row and helps balance out the work done by the pressing muscles.
- **Key tip**: Focus on retracting the scapula at the top of the movement to fully engage the traps and rhomboids. Avoid using too much weight, as this can compromise form and reduce the effectiveness of the exercise.

3. Barbell or Dumbbell Shrugs

Shrugs are an excellent accessory exercise for isolating the upper trapezius muscles, which play a key role in the finishing portion of the bent-over row. Strengthening the traps improves your ability to fully contract and stabilize your upper back during rowing motions.

- **How to do it**: Stand with a barbell or dumbbells at arm's length in front of you. Keep your arms straight, engage your core, and lift your shoulders towards your ears in a shrugging motion. Hold at the top for a second, then slowly lower the weights back to the starting position.
- **When to use it**: Shrugs can be used as part of your accessory routine to enhance the strength of the traps. Stronger traps can help with stabilizing the scapula during bent-over rows and other upper-body movements.
- **Key tip**: Keep your arms relaxed throughout the movement and avoid using your forearms to "pull" the weight. The movement should come entirely from your traps.

4. Single-Arm Dumbbell Row

The single-arm dumbbell row is a great variation of the bent-over row that targets the lats and rhomboids, while also emphasizing unilateral strength. This movement allows you to focus on each side individually, helping to correct any muscle imbalances that might affect your overall rowing technique.

- **How to do it**: Place one knee and hand on a bench for support, with the other foot flat on the floor. With a dumbbell in the free hand, row the weight towards your hip, keeping your elbow close to your body. Squeeze your shoulder blade at the top, then lower the dumbbell back to the starting position.
- **When to use it**: Incorporate single-arm dumbbell rows into your accessory routine to isolate the lats and address any asymmetries in strength between sides.
- **Key tip**: Avoid twisting your torso during the movement, and ensure the motion comes from your back muscles rather than relying on your arm to pull the weight.

5. Inverted Rows

Inverted rows are an excellent bodyweight movement for building pulling strength and improving the activation of the muscles targeted during bent-over rows. They work the entire back, including the lats, traps, rhomboids, and rear delts, and can be scaled based on your strength level.

- **How to do it**: Set up a barbell in a rack at waist height or use a suspension trainer (like TRX). Position your body under the bar, gripping it with both hands. Your body should be in a straight line from head to heels. Pull your chest towards the bar by squeezing your shoulder blades together, then lower yourself back down with control.
- **When to use it**: Inverted rows can serve as a great warm-up or accessory movement to reinforce proper pulling mechanics. They are also a fantastic option if you need to build the basic strength required for heavier rows.
- **Key tip**: Keep your body straight throughout the movement and focus on retracting your scapula. Avoid letting your hips sag or arching your lower back excessively.

6. Hammer Curls

While bent-over rows predominantly target the upper back, hammer curls are an effective accessory exercise to strengthen the forearms and biceps, which assist with grip strength during rowing movements. Stronger forearms and biceps will not only help you hold onto the bar but also improve the quality of your rows by allowing you to pull with greater force.

- **How to do it**: Hold a dumbbell in each hand with a neutral (palms facing in) grip. Keeping your elbows close to your body, curl the dumbbells towards your shoulders, then lower them slowly back to the starting position.
- **When to use it**: Include hammer curls in your accessory routine to improve forearm and bicep strength. These muscles play an important role in maintaining a secure grip during bent-over rows and other pulling exercises.
- **Key tip**: Focus on keeping your upper arms stationary and isolating the movement to your forearms. Don't swing your body or use momentum to lift the weights.

7. Key Flexibility Drills for Improving Range of Motion

Flexibility and mobility are key components of a well-rounded strength program. Improving your range of motion will allow you to execute bent-over rows with proper form, thereby reducing the risk of injury and maximizing muscle engagement.

- **Thoracic Spine Mobility**: Perform foam rolling or mobility drills to improve the flexibility of the thoracic spine (mid-back). This will allow for a better range of motion when retracting the scapula during the row.
- **Hip Flexor and Hamstring Stretching**: Tight hip flexors and hamstrings can limit your ability to properly hinge at the hips during the bent-over row, resulting in poor posture and less effective muscle activation. Incorporate hip stretches to improve your flexibility in these areas.
- **Shoulder Mobility**: Perform shoulder dislocations using a resistance band or broomstick to improve your range of motion in the shoulder joint, which will enhance your ability to perform rows with proper scapular retraction and depression.

Conclusion

Incorporating these accessory movements into your training routine will help to build a strong foundation for your bent-over rows, improving both strength and form. By targeting the lats, traps, rhomboids, biceps, forearms, and shoulders, you'll reinforce the muscles that play a critical role in rowing movements. Whether you're seeking to improve your overall pulling power, prevent imbalances, or increase hypertrophy in your upper body, these accessory exercises will help you achieve your goals and take your strength training to the next level.

Chapter 19: Overcoming Plateaus in the Bent-Over Row

Plateaus are a common hurdle in any strength training program, and the bent-over row is no exception. Whether you're a beginner or an advanced lifter, you will likely experience times when your progress stalls, and the gains you once made seem to plateau. This can be frustrating, but it's a natural part of the training process. Understanding how to identify, manage, and overcome plateaus in the bent-over row can help you break through these barriers and continue progressing toward your strength goals.

In this chapter, we'll explore various strategies for overcoming plateaus in the bent-over row. These strategies focus on adjusting volume, intensity, and exercise variations, as well as addressing any weaknesses or imbalances that may be limiting your progress. By employing these techniques, you can keep your rowing movements fresh, stimulating, and most importantly—effective.

1. Identifying Plateaus: What to Look For

Plateaus occur when the body no longer responds to the same stimulus, and muscle growth or strength gains stall. In the case of the bent-over row, signs that you're facing a plateau may include:

- **Stagnant Weight**: You're no longer able to increase the weight you're lifting, even though you feel you should be able to.
- **Decreased Reps**: You might notice that you're unable to perform the same number of repetitions at a given weight as you once could.
- **Lack of Progress in Assistance Movements**: Even though you're putting in the effort, accessory exercises and supplementary lifts such as lat pulldowns or face pulls are showing little to no improvement.
- **Mental Fatigue**: You may feel unmotivated or bored with your rowing sessions, and the excitement you once had for the exercise is gone.

Recognizing these signs early can help you adjust your training plan before the plateau becomes permanent.

2. Managing Volume and Intensity

One of the primary reasons plateaus happen is a lack of variation in training volume and intensity. Your body adapts to the stimuli you provide, so consistently doing the same number of sets and reps, or lifting the same amount of weight, can cause your progress to stall. To overcome this, consider implementing these changes:

- **Increase Volume Gradually**: If you've been doing the same amount of work for a while, try increasing your weekly volume. This can mean adding an extra set or increasing the number of repetitions per set. A gradual increase in volume can provide a new stimulus that challenges the muscles in a different way.
  Example: If you've been doing 4 sets of 8 reps, try 5 sets of 8-10 reps or increase your rep range to 12 per set for a few weeks.
- **Vary Intensity**: If your strength gains have stalled, it's time to adjust your intensity. This might mean lifting heavier weights for lower reps, or using lighter weights for higher reps, depending on your goal. Additionally, altering rest intervals or adding more explosive movements can help break through a plateau.
  Example: Incorporate low-rep, heavy sets (3-5 reps) for 3-4 sets in one session, and switch to moderate weights with higher reps (10-12 reps) in another session.
- **Change Tempo and Rest Periods**: Slowing down the eccentric (lowering) phase of the lift increases time under tension, which can lead to greater muscle growth. Alternatively, shortening your rest periods can challenge endurance and push the muscles to fatigue faster. Both approaches can reignite progress by adding new stimulus.

3. Targeting Weak Muscle Groups

Plateaus often occur because specific muscles involved in the bent-over row have become the limiting factor. Identifying and strengthening weak muscle groups can lead to improvements in your rowing performance and help break through the plateau.

- **Focus on Grip Strength**: A common limiting factor in the bent-over row is grip strength. If your hands tire before your back muscles, your performance will suffer. Incorporating exercises like dead hangs, farmer's walks, and wrist curls can help build a stronger grip.
  Tip: Use lifting straps if grip strength is a major limiting factor, but only as a temporary measure while you focus on improving grip strength over time.
- **Strengthen Your Lats**: Weak lats can limit your ability to properly execute a bent-over row. If you're struggling to engage your back muscles fully, consider adding lat-focused exercises like lat pulldowns, pull-ups, and single-arm dumbbell rows to your routine.
- **Improve Core Stability**: A weak core can cause you to lose form and limit your ability to generate force through the torso. Strengthening the core through exercises like planks, leg raises, and cable woodchoppers can help maintain stability and improve performance in the bent-over row.

4. Implementing Progressive Variations

One of the most effective ways to overcome a plateau is by changing the stimulus you provide to the muscles. For the bent-over row, this can be achieved through variations in form, grip, and positioning. These variations can target different aspects of the back and help break the stagnation in your progress.

- **T-Bar Rows**: This variation allows you to lift heavier weights and focus on the mid-back, particularly the rhomboids and traps. By incorporating T-bar rows into your routine, you can strengthen the pulling muscles and potentially overload them to break through plateaus.
- **Chest-Supported Rows**: A chest-supported row machine or bench isolates the back muscles by minimizing the involvement of other muscles such as the lower back and hamstrings. This variation can be particularly helpful if you're experiencing lower back fatigue during bent-over rows.
- **Single-Arm Dumbbell Rows**: Single-arm rows allow you to isolate each side of your back, which can help address any imbalances that may exist between your left and right sides. This can also provide a greater range of motion, which can enhance overall muscle development.
- **Pendlay Rows**: This variation involves pulling the bar from the floor with every rep, which helps to emphasize explosive power and lower back activation. Pendlay rows are a great way to introduce speed and power into your rowing movements, which can help break through plateaus.

5. Incorporating Deload Weeks

If you've been pushing hard for several weeks without seeing improvement, it may be time to introduce a deload week. A deload week involves reducing the intensity, volume, or both, to allow your body to recover and reset. This brief break can give your muscles and nervous system the chance to fully recover, leading to improved performance when you resume training.

How to Implement

6. Mental Strategies: Breaking Through the Mental Barrier

Sometimes, a plateau isn't just about physical adaptation but mental fatigue. Strength training can become monotonous, and the excitement of hitting new personal records can fade. To combat this, you can incorporate some mental strategies:

- **Visualization**: Imagine yourself executing the perfect bent-over row with good form and feeling strong. This mental practice can increase your confidence and help you push past mental barriers in the gym.
- **Goal Setting**: Reassess your goals and set both short-term and long-term objectives for your training. Breaking your progress into achievable steps can keep you motivated and focused.
- **Accountability**: Whether it's a training partner or a coach, having someone hold you accountable for your performance can help you stay on track and prevent you from becoming complacent.

Conclusion

Plateaus in strength training, especially in exercises like the bent-over row, are a natural part of the process. While they can be frustrating, they also present an opportunity to reevaluate your training strategies and make the necessary adjustments to continue progressing. By managing volume and intensity, addressing weak muscle groups, implementing variations, incorporating deload weeks, and using mental strategies, you can overcome plateaus and keep making progress toward your strength goals. Stay consistent, stay focused, and remember that breaking through plateaus is not just about lifting more weight—it's about smart training and continuous improvement.

Chapter 20: Advanced Bent-Over Row Techniques

The bent-over row is a foundational movement that targets the back, primarily working the latissimus dorsi, rhomboids, traps, and biceps. However, as you advance in strength training, simply performing the basic bent-over row may not provide enough stimulus to continue progressing. To break through plateaus, increase muscle mass, and enhance overall pulling power, it's essential to explore advanced row variations, targeting different angles and muscle groups. In this chapter, we'll explore several advanced techniques to take your bent-over row to the next level, ensuring balanced back development and improved pulling strength.

1. T-Bar Rows: Targeting the Mid and Upper Back

T-Bar rows are an advanced variation that isolates the mid-back and traps while allowing you to lift heavier weights compared to the standard barbell row. This exercise emphasizes horizontal pulling and helps to build thickness and power in the back, especially the rhomboids and middle traps.

- **How to do it**: Set up a T-Bar row machine or landmine attachment. Position yourself with your feet shoulder-width apart and knees slightly bent. Grip the handles or bar with a pronated (overhand) grip and pull the weight towards your torso, keeping your elbows close to your body. Focus on retracting your shoulder blades at the top of the movement and squeezing your mid-back.
- **When to use it**: T-Bar rows are excellent for building back thickness and targeting the rhomboids and traps. Incorporate them into your back training routine to vary the angle of your pulls and provide a new stimulus to your muscles.
- **Key tip**: Keep your back straight and avoid using momentum to pull the weight. The movement should come from your back muscles rather than your arms or lower back.

2. Chest-Supported Rows: Reducing Lower Back Fatigue

Chest-supported rows are a variation that eliminates the need for lower back stabilization, allowing you to isolate the back muscles more effectively. This exercise helps to remove the strain on the lower back, which can be a limiting factor in the traditional bent-over row.

- **How to do it**: Set up a chest-supported row machine or use an incline bench to support your chest. Grip the handles or a barbell with a neutral or overhand grip. Pull the weight towards your chest while keeping your elbows close to your body. Squeeze your shoulder blades together at the top of the movement, then slowly lower the weight back to the starting position.
- **When to use it**: Chest-supported rows are useful when you want to isolate the upper back without compromising lower back stability. These can be a great option for lifters who struggle with maintaining proper posture during bent-over rows due to lower back fatigue.
- **Key tip**: Focus on keeping a controlled motion throughout the set. Don't allow your body to move or your chest to lift off the bench. Maintain a strong, steady pull using your back muscles.

3. Single-Arm Dumbbell Rows: Isolating Each Side for Balanced Strength

Single-arm dumbbell rows allow you to isolate each side of the back, which can help address muscle imbalances and improve unilateral strength. This movement also provides a greater range of motion compared to the traditional barbell row, allowing for a deeper stretch and contraction in the lats.

- **How to do it**: Place one knee and hand on a bench, creating a stable position. With the opposite hand, grab a dumbbell and row it towards your torso. Focus on driving the elbow back and squeezing the shoulder blade at the top of the movement. Lower the dumbbell with control and repeat for the desired number of reps.
- **When to use it**: Single-arm rows are excellent for targeting the lats and improving symmetry in the back. They're also ideal for lifters who experience difficulty engaging one side of their back during barbell rows.
- **Key tip**: Ensure that your torso remains stable throughout the movement. Avoid rotating your body or using momentum to lift the weight. The movement should come solely from your back muscles.

4. Barbell Rows from the Floor (Pendlay Rows)

Pendlay rows are a variation that emphasizes explosiveness and power by lifting the barbell from a dead stop on the floor with each repetition. This variation engages more of the posterior chain, including the lower back, hamstrings, and glutes, while building explosive strength in the lats and upper back.

- **How to do it**: Set the barbell on the floor with a loaded weight, and stand with your feet shoulder-width apart. Bend at the hips and knees to grip the bar with an overhand grip, slightly wider than shoulder-width. In one fluid motion, pull the bar explosively towards your chest, keeping your back flat and your core engaged. Lower the bar back to the floor, ensuring it comes to a complete stop before starting the next rep.
- **When to use it**: Pendlay rows are great for developing explosive pulling power, especially in athletes who need to improve their dynamic strength. They also help reinforce proper deadlift positioning and hip hinge mechanics.
- **Key tip**: Focus on driving through your heels and keeping your chest up throughout the movement. Avoid rounding your back, as this can increase the risk of injury.

5. Renegade Rows: Combining Core Stability with Upper-Body Strength

Renegade rows are a full-body movement that combines a plank with a rowing motion, requiring core stability and upper-body strength. This exercise is great for developing back strength while also engaging the core and improving coordination.

- **How to do it**: Start in a push-up position with a dumbbell in each hand. Row one dumbbell towards your torso while maintaining a stable plank position. Lower the dumbbell back to the floor and repeat on the other side. Make sure to engage your core throughout the movement to prevent your hips from rotating.
- **When to use it**: Renegade rows can be used as an accessory movement to improve core stability and back strength. They are also an excellent option for those looking to incorporate functional, compound movements into their workout.
- **Key tip**: Keep your body as still as possible while performing the row, avoiding any twisting or swaying of the hips. Engage your core to maintain a stable plank position.

6. Seated Cable Rows: Focusing on Back Width and Detail

Seated cable rows are a great accessory movement for adding variety to your rowing routine. By adjusting the grip and cable attachment, you can target different parts of the back and vary the stimulus placed on the muscles.

- **How to do it**: Sit at a cable row machine with your feet planted firmly and knees slightly bent. Grip the handle with a neutral or pronated grip, keeping your arms extended in front of you. Pull the handle towards your torso, focusing on squeezing the shoulder blades together. Keep your chest up and avoid leaning backward excessively during the movement.
- **When to use it**: Seated cable rows are excellent for targeting the lats and mid-back. By adjusting the grip, you can focus on different angles of the back for balanced development. They can be a great complement to your heavy bent-over rows.
- **Key tip**: Focus on pulling with your back muscles, not your arms. Keep the movement smooth and controlled, with a strong squeeze at the end of each repetition.

7. Integrating Rows with Other Pulling Exercises

To develop a truly powerful back, it's essential to integrate the bent-over row with other pulling exercises. These can include vertical pulling movements such as pull-ups and lat pulldowns, as well as horizontal pulling movements like chest-supported rows or face pulls. Combining different angles and types of pulls ensures balanced muscle development and improves overall back strength.

- **How to do it**: Incorporate a variety of pulling movements into your weekly routine. For example, pair bent-over rows with pull-ups or lat pulldowns for a balanced approach to building back strength. You can also alternate between different rowing variations throughout the week to prevent adaptation and promote muscle growth.
- **When to use it**: Use a combination of pulling exercises to ensure all areas of the back are targeted. This approach will lead to more comprehensive back development and enhanced pulling power.
- **Key tip**: Don't neglect accessory exercises like face pulls and rear delt work, as they play a crucial role in shoulder health and overall upper-body strength.

Conclusion

Advanced bent-over row techniques are essential for breaking through plateaus and continuing to develop back strength, hypertrophy, and overall pulling power. Whether you're targeting the mid-back with T-Bar rows, isolating one side with single-arm dumbbell rows, or adding explosive power with Pendlay rows, these variations will help keep your training dynamic and effective. By incorporating different angles, grips, and accessory exercises into your routine, you can maximize your back development and build a stronger, more powerful body. Keep experimenting with these advanced techniques to continually challenge yourself and push the boundaries of your strength.

Chapter 21: Designing a Complete Strength Training Program

Designing a strength training program that incorporates the bench press, military press, and bent-over rows is crucial for achieving balanced, total-body strength and performance. Whether you're a beginner or an advanced lifter, structuring a routine that combines compound lifts, accessory exercises, and adequate recovery is key to making consistent progress. In this chapter, we will explore how to create a comprehensive training program that targets all major muscle groups, ensures proper recovery, and allows for progressive overload to maximize strength gains.

1. Understanding the Importance of a Balanced Program

A well-rounded strength training program should consist of three main components:

- **Compound movements** like the bench press, military press, and bent-over row, which work multiple muscle groups simultaneously and form the foundation of strength training.
- **Accessory movements** to address muscle imbalances, improve joint health, and target secondary muscles that support the compound lifts.
- **Recovery** to ensure muscles repair and grow stronger after each session.

By combining these elements, you create a holistic program that not only develops strength but also promotes muscle growth, mobility, and injury prevention.

2. Structuring Your Weekly Plan

When structuring your training week, the goal is to balance the intensity, volume, and frequency of your workouts to avoid overtraining while ensuring continued progress. A typical program will feature 3-5 training days per week, with varying focuses to allow for muscle recovery and optimal performance.

Beginner Program (3 Days per Week)

- **Day 1:** Bench Press, Military Press, Bent-Over Rows, Accessory Chest and Shoulder Movements
- **Day 2:** Lower Body (Squats, Deadlifts, Lunges)
- **Day 3:** Bench Press, Military Press, Bent-Over Rows, Accessory Back and Arm Movements

Intermediate Program (4 Days per Week)

- **Day 1:** Upper Body (Bench Press, Military Press, Bent-Over Rows, Triceps, Shoulders)
- **Day 2:** Lower Body (Squats, Deadlifts, Hamstring Work)
- **Day 3:** Upper Body (Accessory Rows, Chest, Biceps, Core)
- **Day 4:** Lower Body (Lunges, Deadlifts, Glute and Calf Work)

Advanced Program (5 Days per Week)

- **Day 1:** Chest and Shoulders (Bench Press, Military Press, Chest Accessory)
- **Day 2:** Back and Biceps (Bent-Over Rows, Pull-Ups, Arm Movements)
- **Day 3:** Legs (Squats, Deadlifts, Leg Press)
- **Day 4:** Full Upper Body (Accessory Movements for Shoulders, Back, Chest)
- **Day 5:** Full Body or Specialization (Power Movements, Heavy Rows or Presses)

3. Combining Compound and Accessory Exercises

While the bench press, military press, and bent-over rows are the cornerstones of your program, it's essential to include accessory lifts that support these movements and enhance overall strength. These exercises help to improve stability, target secondary muscle groups, and correct muscle imbalances.

Accessory lifts for the bench press:

- **Triceps dips**: Focus on strengthening the triceps, which play a crucial role in the lockout phase of the bench press.
- **Chest flys**: Target the chest more directly, providing hypertrophy in the pectorals.
- **Shoulder stability exercises**: To help maintain shoulder health, exercises like face pulls and rotator cuff work are key.

Accessory lifts for the military press:

- **Lateral raises**: Strengthen the lateral deltoids, improving the overall shoulder structure and helping with pressing power.
- **Triceps extensions**: Focus on developing triceps strength, which is crucial for a strong lockout during the press.
- **Face pulls**: Strengthen the rear delts and improve shoulder health for pressing motions.

Accessory lifts for the bent-over row:

- **Lat pull-downs**: A vertical pull variation that targets the lats to complement horizontal pulling movements.
- **Single-arm dumbbell rows**: Work each side of the back independently to correct muscle imbalances.
- **Trap work**: Shrugs and upright rows can help strengthen the upper traps, which contribute to the stability of the shoulder girdle during rowing.

By combining these compound lifts with accessory movements, you'll not only enhance strength but also help prevent injury and imbalances that can result from focusing on the big lifts alone.

4. Frequency, Volume, and Intensity Recommendations

For optimal progress, it's essential to tailor your training based on your experience level. The following recommendations provide guidelines on frequency, volume, and intensity for each experience level.

Beginners

- **Frequency**: 3 training sessions per week
- **Volume**: 3-4 sets of 8-12 reps for most exercises
- **Intensity**: Start with light to moderate weight, focusing on form and technique
- **Rest**: 1-2 minutes between sets

Intermediate Lifters

- **Frequency**: 4 training sessions per week
- **Volume**: 4-5 sets of 5-8 reps for compound movements, 8-12 reps for accessory lifts
- **Intensity**: Use moderate to heavy weights (70-85% of 1RM)
- **Rest**: 2-3 minutes between sets for compound lifts, 1-2 minutes for accessory exercises

Advanced Lifters

- **Frequency**: 4-5 training sessions per week
- **Volume**: 4-6 sets of 3-6 reps for compound lifts, 6-12 reps for accessory movements
- **Intensity**: Train with heavy weights (85-95% of 1RM), using advanced techniques like drop sets and supersets
- **Rest**: 3-4 minutes between sets for compound lifts, 1-2 minutes for accessory lifts

5. Rest, Recovery, and Deloading Strategies

To achieve the best results, your body needs time to recover and adapt to the stresses placed upon it during training. Overtraining can lead to injuries and hinder progress, so incorporating rest and recovery into your program is essential.

- **Rest Days**: Schedule at least 1-2 rest days per week to allow your muscles to recover. On rest days, focus on light activity like walking, stretching, or yoga to promote blood circulation and flexibility.
- **Sleep**: Aim for 7-9 hours of quality sleep each night to ensure your body has the opportunity to repair and grow muscle tissue.
- **Deload Weeks**: Every 4-8 weeks, incorporate a deload week, where you reduce the intensity and volume of your workouts to allow the body to fully recover. This is particularly important for advanced lifters who often push the intensity and may risk burnout or injury.

During a deload week, you may reduce weights by 50-60% and lower the volume to 2-3 sets per exercise. Focus on technique and mobility work rather than pushing for new personal records.

6. Tracking Progress and Adjusting Your Program

Tracking your progress is essential for ensuring that you're continuously moving toward your goals. Keep a training log that includes the following:

- **Exercises performed**
- **Sets, reps, and weights used**
- **Rest intervals**
- **Notes on how you felt during the workout**

Review your progress weekly or monthly to assess improvements in strength, muscle growth, and performance. If you hit a plateau, adjust your routine by changing the rep ranges, switching accessory exercises, or focusing on improving form and technique.

Conclusion

Designing a comprehensive strength training program is the key to achieving total power and performance. By structuring your weekly routine around the bench press, military press, and bent-over rows, and complementing them with accessory movements, you can target all the major muscle groups, increase strength, and prevent imbalances. Incorporating proper recovery strategies and adjusting the program as needed will ensure long-term success. Remember, the journey of strength mastery is a marathon, not a sprint—consistency, patience, and progression are the cornerstones of achieving your goals.

Chapter 22: Nutrition for Strength and Performance

Strength training and proper nutrition are deeply interconnected. What you eat before, during, and after your workouts can significantly impact your performance, recovery, and overall muscle growth. This chapter will delve into the essential nutrients required for strength development, how to time your meals, and the role of hydration in supporting optimal performance. Whether you're a beginner or an advanced lifter, understanding how nutrition impacts your strength goals is essential for achieving total power and performance.

1. The Role of Protein, Carbohydrates, and Fats in Strength Training

To support muscle growth, repair, and performance, you need to provide your body with the right nutrients. Each macronutrient—protein, carbohydrates, and fats—plays a unique role in fueling your workouts and helping your body recover.

Protein: The Building Block of Muscle

- **Importance**: Protein is essential for muscle repair and growth. During strength training, muscle fibers undergo small tears, and protein helps to rebuild and strengthen them.
- **How Much Do You Need?**: The general recommendation for strength athletes is 1.6 to 2.2 grams of protein per kilogram of body weight (0.7-1 gram per pound). For example, a 180-pound (82 kg) individual would aim for about 130-180 grams of protein per day.
- **Sources**: Lean meats (chicken, turkey, lean beef), fish, eggs, dairy, legumes, and plant-based protein sources like tofu and tempeh are excellent choices.

Carbohydrates: Your Fuel Source

- **Importance**: Carbohydrates are the primary source of energy for high-intensity workouts. Without adequate carbs, your body will struggle to fuel your muscles, reducing your workout intensity and increasing fatigue.
- **How Much Do You Need?**: Carbohydrate needs vary depending on the volume and intensity of your training, but strength athletes should aim for about 3-7 grams of carbohydrates per kilogram of body weight, with more carbs needed on high-intensity training days.
- **Sources**: Whole grains (brown rice, oats, quinoa), fruits, vegetables, and legumes are great options that provide sustained energy.

Fats: Hormonal Health and Energy

- **Importance**: Healthy fats are crucial for maintaining hormonal balance, particularly for testosterone and growth hormone, which are vital for muscle growth. Fats also provide a slow-burning source of energy for long workouts or recovery periods.
- **How Much Do You Need?**: About 20-35% of your total daily caloric intake should come from fats, with an emphasis on unsaturated fats.
- **Sources**: Avocados, olive oil, nuts, seeds, fatty fish (salmon, mackerel), and coconut oil are excellent sources of healthy fats.

2. Meal Timing and Supplementation

What you eat and when you eat it can have a major impact on your performance, recovery, and muscle-building potential. Strategic meal timing ensures that your body has the necessary nutrients for energy and muscle repair when it needs them most.

Pre-Workout Nutrition: Fueling for Performance

- **Timing**: Consume a balanced meal 1-2 hours before your workout. This meal should include a mix of carbohydrates, protein, and a small amount of fats to provide steady energy.
- **Ideal Foods**: A piece of whole-grain toast with almond butter and banana, or oatmeal with protein powder, is an excellent choice.
- **Why It Matters**: Carbohydrates provide the energy needed for strength training, while protein ensures that muscles have amino acids available to prevent breakdown during the workout.

Post-Workout Nutrition: Maximizing Recovery

- **Timing**: Aim to eat a protein-rich meal within 30-60 minutes after training to kickstart muscle recovery. This is when your body is most receptive to nutrient uptake.
- **Ideal Foods**: A protein shake with a carb source (such as a banana or a piece of toast) is perfect for post-workout. Alternatively, a meal like grilled chicken with sweet potatoes and vegetables is another excellent option.
- **Why It Matters**: After lifting, muscles are in a catabolic state and need protein to rebuild. Carbs help replenish muscle glycogen stores, ensuring you're ready for your next workout.

General Meal Timing Tips

- Eat 4-6 smaller meals throughout the day to maintain energy levels and promote steady muscle growth.
- Stay consistent with meal timing to help regulate your body's nutrient absorption and muscle repair processes.

Supplements for Strength Training

- **Whey Protein**: A quick and easy way to meet your protein needs, especially post-workout.
- **Creatine**: One of the most researched supplements, creatine helps increase strength, improve power output, and reduce fatigue during high-intensity exercises.
- **Branched-Chain Amino Acids (BCAAs)**: These can reduce muscle soreness and help prevent muscle breakdown during prolonged or intense training sessions.
- **Beta-Alanine**: This supplement helps buffer lactic acid buildup, reducing fatigue during high-repetition or high-intensity workouts.
- **Fish Oil**: Omega-3 fatty acids help with joint health, reduce inflammation, and support overall recovery.

3. Hydration and Its Impact on Performance

Hydration is an often overlooked yet critical factor for strength training success. Dehydration can impair strength, endurance, and focus, leading to subpar performance and a higher risk of injury.

How Much Water Do You Need?

- A general guideline is to drink at least 3.7 liters (125 ounces) of water daily for men and 2.7 liters (91 ounces) for women. However, this can vary depending on climate, workout intensity, and body size.
- **Pre-Workout Hydration**: Drink 16-20 ounces of water 1-2 hours before training to ensure optimal hydration.
- **During Workout Hydration**: Aim to drink 7-10 ounces of water every 10-20 minutes during exercise, particularly in hot environments or during long sessions.
- **Post-Workout Hydration**: Replenish lost fluids with at least 16-24 ounces of water following exercise. Consider adding electrolytes to help restore sodium, potassium, and other vital minerals.

Electrolytes and Sports Drinks

Sports drinks or electrolyte tablets are particularly useful for endurance athletes but can also benefit strength athletes during prolonged sessions or intense workouts.

4. Special Considerations for Strength Athletes

While general nutrition principles apply to everyone, strength athletes have specific needs that should be considered to maximize performance and muscle development.

Caloric Surplus vs. Caloric Deficit

- **Building Muscle (Caloric Surplus)**: If your goal is to build muscle, you'll need to eat in a slight caloric surplus. This means consuming more calories than your body burns to support muscle growth and recovery.
- **Cutting Fat (Caloric Deficit)**: If you're focusing on fat loss while preserving strength, aim for a slight caloric deficit, making sure to maintain a high protein intake to prevent muscle loss.

Meal Composition Based on Training Days

- **Training Days**: On workout days, emphasize carbohydrate intake around your training window to ensure you have sufficient energy for your lifts and promote muscle recovery afterward.
- **Rest Days**: On non-training days, you may slightly reduce carbohydrate intake but maintain protein intake to preserve muscle mass.

5. Conclusion

Nutrition is a cornerstone of strength training success. By properly fueling your body with the right balance of protein, carbohydrates, fats, and hydration, you can maximize your strength, recovery, and performance. Strategic meal timing, supplementation, and adequate hydration are key to ensuring that your body has the energy and nutrients needed to power through your workouts and recover efficiently. With the right nutritional plan, you can optimize your training and take your strength to new heights.

Chapter 23: Recovery: The Key to Growth

In the pursuit of strength and performance, recovery is often the most overlooked component. Training hard and pushing yourself to lift heavier, perform more reps, or go for longer durations is essential, but without adequate recovery, all that effort can be wasted. This chapter will explore the vital role recovery plays in building strength and muscle mass, as well as effective strategies to help your body repair, grow, and prepare for your next session.

1. Sleep and Its Impact on Muscle Growth

Sleep is arguably the most important recovery tool you have, yet it is frequently neglected. Quality sleep is when your body undergoes the majority of its repair processes, including muscle growth and tissue regeneration. Without sufficient rest, your muscles cannot fully recover, and performance gains are diminished.

- **Muscle Recovery and Growth**: During deep sleep, growth hormone levels rise, stimulating muscle tissue repair and promoting protein synthesis. This is crucial after intense strength training, which causes microscopic tears in muscle fibers. Recovery allows these fibers to rebuild stronger and larger.
- **Sleep Duration**: Strength athletes should aim for 7-9 hours of sleep per night. Some individuals may require more sleep during heavy training cycles, while others might find 7 hours sufficient. Listening to your body's needs is key.
- **Sleep Quality**: It's not just about how much you sleep, but how well you sleep. Poor sleep quality can interfere with muscle recovery and leave you feeling fatigued during workouts. To improve sleep quality:

- Maintain a regular sleep schedule (even on weekends).
- Avoid caffeine, nicotine, and heavy meals close to bedtime.
- Create a cool, dark, and quiet sleep environment.
- Limit screen time before bed to enhance melatonin production.

Napping for Extra Recovery

2. Stretching, Foam Rolling, and Mobility Work

Although strength training is critical for building muscle, flexibility and mobility are essential for joint health and performance. Incorporating stretching and foam rolling into your recovery routine can reduce muscle tightness, improve flexibility, and prevent injury.

Stretching

- **Static Stretching**: Performed after workouts, static stretching involves holding a stretch for 20-30 seconds, targeting tight muscle groups to improve flexibility.
- **Dynamic Stretching**: Dynamic stretches, such as leg swings or arm circles, are best performed before workouts to warm up muscles and prepare them for the demands of lifting.

Foam Rolling

Focus on key areas such as the lower back, quads, hamstrings, and calves. Spend 1-2 minutes on each area, but avoid rolling directly over joints or bones.

Mobility Work

Incorporate mobility drills like hip openers, shoulder rotations, and ankle dorsiflexion into your recovery routine to maintain proper posture and prevent movement dysfunction.

3. Active Recovery and Low-Intensity Exercise

While complete rest days are important, active recovery can also aid in muscle repair. Low-intensity exercise boosts blood circulation, which accelerates the delivery of nutrients and removal of waste products from muscles, aiding in the recovery process.

Active Recovery Ideas

- **Light Cardio**: A brisk walk, light cycling, or swimming can stimulate circulation without putting stress on the muscles. Aim for 20-30 minutes of steady-state cardio at an easy pace.
- **Yoga**: Yoga improves flexibility, reduces muscle stiffness, and promotes relaxation. Many yoga poses, such as downward dog, child's pose, and cat-cow, are excellent for loosening up tight muscles.
- **Swimming**: Swimming is a great full-body exercise that promotes blood flow and provides low-impact movement for recovery, especially for individuals with joint or muscle pain.

Rest Days

4. Nutrition and Supplementation for Recovery

Nutrition plays an integral role in muscle repair and recovery. After strength training, your muscles need the right nutrients to rebuild and grow stronger. Ensuring proper post-workout nutrition is key to maximizing recovery.

- **Protein**: Consuming a protein-rich meal or shake within 30-60 minutes after a workout helps stimulate muscle protein synthesis and accelerate muscle repair. Aim for 20-40 grams of high-quality protein from sources like whey protein, chicken, turkey, fish, or plant-based protein powders.
- **Carbohydrates**: After a workout, muscle glycogen stores (the body's stored form of carbohydrate) are depleted. Eating carbohydrates after training helps replenish these stores, ensuring you have energy for your next session. Choose complex carbs such as sweet potatoes, quinoa, brown rice, and oats.
- **Healthy Fats**: Fats are important for overall recovery, especially for joint health and hormone production. Incorporate healthy fats like avocados, olive oil, nuts, and seeds into your meals.
- **Hydration**: Rehydrating after a workout is vital to restoring fluid balance, as dehydration can slow recovery. Drink water throughout the day, and consider a post-workout electrolyte drink to replace sodium, potassium, and other minerals lost in sweat.
- **Supplements for Recovery**:

- **BCAAs (Branched-Chain Amino Acids)**: BCAAs may help reduce muscle soreness and prevent muscle breakdown during recovery.
- **Creatine**: While primarily used to enhance performance, creatine also plays a role in muscle recovery by supporting ATP production during training.
- **Glutamine**: This amino acid helps with muscle recovery and immune function, particularly after intense workouts.
- **Fish Oil**: Omega-3 fatty acids from fish oil have anti-inflammatory properties, helping reduce muscle soreness and promote joint health.

5. Avoiding Overtraining and Preventing Injury

While it's crucial to push your limits in the gym, it's equally important to listen to your body and avoid overtraining. Overtraining occurs when the body does not have enough time to recover between sessions, which can lead to diminished performance, fatigue, and an increased risk of injury.

- **Signs of Overtraining**: These include persistent fatigue, irritability, difficulty sleeping, decreased performance, increased soreness, and a weakened immune system. If you experience any of these symptoms, it's essential to take a step back, reduce training intensity, and prioritize recovery.
- **Preventing Injury**: Proper recovery strategies help to prevent overuse injuries, which are common when training too hard without proper rest. Incorporate regular mobility work, stretching, and foam rolling to maintain flexibility and joint health. Always use proper form and technique during lifts to avoid strain on muscles and ligaments.

6. Conclusion

Recovery is where the magic happens. Strength gains don't occur while you're lifting weights—they occur during the recovery process. Adequate sleep, nutrition, stretching, foam rolling, and active recovery are essential components for muscle repair and growth. By prioritizing recovery and avoiding overtraining, you can improve performance, prevent injuries, and continue making progress toward your strength goals. Treat recovery as part of your training program, and you'll reap the benefits of enhanced performance, greater strength, and long-term success.

Chapter 24: Mental Toughness in Strength Training

Mental toughness is the often-overlooked ingredient that separates those who simply lift weights from those who truly build strength. The ability to push through physical discomfort, to maintain focus when your muscles are burning, and to continue striving for improvement when progress seems slow or plateaued is what defines a successful strength training journey. This chapter explores how to cultivate mental toughness and integrate it into your training regimen, ensuring that your mind and body are aligned for maximum strength development.

1. Building Resilience and Focus in the Gym

Training for strength is as much a mental challenge as it is a physical one. When you push your body to its limits, your mind plays a pivotal role in determining whether you succeed or fail. Developing resilience allows you to endure setbacks and stay focused on your long-term goals.

- **Resilience Through Repetition**: The process of strength training involves constant progression. At times, you may feel frustrated with slow gains or occasional setbacks. Resilience is developed by accepting these plateaus as a natural part of the process and pushing forward with a positive mindset. Each repetition is an opportunity to grow not only your muscles but also your ability to stay the course.

- **Focus Amid Discomfort**: Strength training is inherently uncomfortable, especially during heavy lifts. Your ability to focus during these moments is what can make or break your performance. The key to maintaining focus is anchoring your mind on the task at hand rather than the discomfort you may be feeling. Concentrating on your breathing, the movement pattern, and your posture can distract you from the pain and keep your body moving effectively.

- **Setting Micro-Goals**: Rather than focusing solely on the big picture, break down your larger goals into smaller, more achievable micro-goals. For example, if you're working to increase your bench press, set a micro-goal of adding 2.5kg to your lift every week. These smaller goals help maintain motivation and provide clear milestones for success.

2. Visualization Techniques and Setting Mental Goals

Visualization is a powerful mental technique that can enhance your performance in the gym. By mentally rehearsing a lift before performing it, you can prepare both your body and mind for the task ahead.

- **Visualization**: Close your eyes and mentally picture yourself performing the lift with perfect form. Visualize the movement in detail—from setting up your body to the path of the barbell and the muscles firing. This process helps create neural pathways that enhance your muscle memory and boost your confidence.

- **Positive Self-Talk**: Your internal dialogue has a significant impact on your performance. If you tell yourself "I can't do this," your body will often follow that suggestion. Alternatively, by adopting a positive mindset and using affirmations like "I am strong, I will push through," you reframe challenges as opportunities to demonstrate your strength.

- **Goal Setting**: Mental toughness thrives on clear and achievable goals. Start with a long-term vision (e.g., hitting a 200kg deadlift) and break it down into smaller, incremental goals (e.g., increasing your deadlift by 5kg every month). Set specific, measurable, achievable, relevant, and time-bound (SMART) goals, and track your progress.

- **Focus on the Process**: Rather than obsessing over the final outcome, embrace the journey of strength building. Focus on the work you're doing in the moment, whether it's your form, technique, or daily training efforts. A process-oriented mindset helps you stay motivated during tough times and reminds you that every session contributes to your overall success.

3. Strategies to Push Through Fatigue and Discomfort

Strength training pushes your body to its limits, and there will inevitably be times when fatigue sets in. The difference between a lifter who stops and one who keeps going often comes down to mental fortitude. Here are some strategies to push through those moments of discomfort:

- **The 5-Second Rule**: The moment you feel resistance—whether physical or mental—your mind may tell you to quit. Use the 5-second rule: when you feel yourself hesitate, count down from five and then act immediately. This can short-circuit hesitation and prevent you from talking yourself out of completing the lift.
- **The "One More Rep" Mentality**: Strength training requires you to push beyond comfort. If you're on your last set and your muscles are screaming, remind yourself to perform just one more rep. That "one more" mentality can often lead to breakthroughs, as it gets you to push past perceived limits and enter a new realm of strength.
- **Embrace the "Fight or Flight" Response**: When facing a tough set, your body will experience an increased heart rate, adrenaline release, and heightened awareness. These natural responses can be harnessed for better performance. Instead of seeing these physiological changes as signals to quit, embrace them as tools to boost your energy and increase your mental toughness.
- **Disassociation**: When you're deep into a tough set and the pain is overwhelming, it can help to disassociate from the discomfort. Focus on your form, your breathing, or the sound of the barbell moving in and out of its path. This mental trick allows you to push through the discomfort by redirecting your mind away from the pain.

4. Developing a Routine for Mental Resilience

Mental toughness is a skill that can be cultivated with practice, much like your physical strength. By establishing a routine that nurtures mental fortitude, you can train your mind to endure the challenges of strength training.

- **Pre-Workout Routine**: The mindset you bring into the gym can greatly impact your performance. Start each session with a mental warm-up, which could involve setting an intention for the workout, reviewing your goals, and doing a brief visualization of your lifts. By creating a consistent pre-workout ritual, you prime your mind for success.
- **Post-Workout Reflection**: After each session, take a few moments to reflect on what you did well and where you can improve. This reflection process helps you mentally process the session and solidifies your learning, while also reinforcing your growth. Use this time to focus on the progress you've made, no matter how small.
- **Resilience Training in Other Areas**: Mental toughness is not limited to the gym. Practice pushing through discomfort in other aspects of life—whether in work, relationships, or personal challenges. The more you practice resilience in various contexts, the stronger your mental toughness becomes.

5. Conclusion

Mental toughness is not something you are born with; it's a quality you can develop over time through consistent effort, practice, and commitment. By learning to manage discomfort, focus on your goals, and visualize success, you'll enhance your strength training experience and unlock your true potential. Developing resilience and mental focus will not only improve your performance in the gym but will carry over to all areas of life. So, the next time you're faced with a challenging set or a tough training day, remember: strength is as much a mental game as it is a physical one. Embrace the struggle, stay focused on the process, and watch your power and performance grow.

Chapter 25: Tracking Progress and Adjusting for Long-Term Success

Strength training is not just about lifting heavier weights or pushing yourself harder every session—it's about consistent, methodical progress over time. To achieve long-term success, you need to track your progress, assess what's working, and adapt your strategy accordingly. This chapter will guide you through the key components of tracking your strength gains, evaluating your progress, and adjusting your routine to continue improving year after year.

1. How to Monitor Your Strength Gains

Tracking your strength gains is essential for staying motivated, ensuring you're making progress, and identifying areas that need improvement. Without measurement, progress can be difficult to assess, and you risk stagnation or burnout. Here are some effective ways to monitor your progress:

- **Record Your Lifts**: Keep a workout journal or use a training app to log every session. Record the weight, sets, and reps for each of your core lifts—the bench press, military press, and bent-over rows—as well as any accessory movements. This will help you track incremental progress and make adjustments to your program.

- **Track Strength Gains Over Time**: In addition to tracking individual workouts, it's essential to assess your overall strength development on a broader scale. Take note of any increase in the maximum weight you can lift for a given exercise or the number of reps you can perform at a specific weight. Set periodic benchmarks to check your progress—e.g., monthly or quarterly.

- **Use Percentage-Based Progression**: Another method for tracking progress is percentage-based tracking. Start with a baseline (e.g., your 1-rep max or a moderate working weight) and track increases as a percentage. For example, if you bench press 100kg for 5 reps, and then later you bench 105kg for the same number of reps, you've made a 5% improvement.

- **Non-Strength Metrics**: Strength gains aren't just about how much you can lift; they also involve improvements in muscle mass, endurance, and recovery. Take regular body measurements and track weight, body fat percentage, and muscle circumference. This will provide a fuller picture of your progress and give you more data to fine-tune your program.

2. Adapting Your Routine as You Progress

As you make gains in your strength training, your body will adapt. Eventually, you may notice that your progress slows or even stalls. This is a natural part of the training process and is known as a "plateau." The key to overcoming plateaus and continuing to progress is knowing when and how to adjust your routine.

- **Increase Intensity**: One of the most effective ways to break through a plateau is to increase the intensity of your lifts. This could mean adding weight, increasing the number of sets or reps, or reducing rest periods between sets to increase training density. Always increase intensity gradually to avoid injury and maintain proper form.

- **Periodization**: Periodization is the practice of varying your training intensity and volume over time. You can divide your program into phases (e.g., strength, hypertrophy, power, recovery) to ensure you're always challenging your body in different ways. For example, after several weeks of heavy lifting, you might shift to a lighter phase that focuses on higher reps to build muscle endurance before returning to heavy, low-rep training.

- **Change Your Training Variables**: If you've been focusing on one rep range (e.g., 3–5 reps for strength), consider switching to a different rep scheme (e.g., 6–8 reps for hypertrophy or 10–12 for endurance). You could also modify other variables such as tempo, rest periods, or exercise variations to continue progressing.

- **Deloading**: Incorporating planned deloads into your routine is crucial for avoiding burnout and overtraining. A deload is a brief period (typically a week) where you reduce the intensity of your training by decreasing the weight, volume, or both. This allows your body to recover and come back stronger for the next phase of training.

- **Accessory Movements**: If you find that your progress in the bench press, military press, or bent-over row has plateaued, incorporating targeted accessory movements can help. For instance, if your bench press is stalling, you might add exercises that strengthen the triceps (e.g., skull crushers or tricep dips) or the shoulders (e.g., dumbbell shoulder press) to break through the sticking point.

3. Tips for Setting and Achieving New Goals Year After Year

The most successful strength athletes don't just set goals—they set goals that are challenging, measurable, and adaptable. As you make progress, it's important to recalibrate your goals regularly to ensure that you're always working toward something that will push you to improve. Here's how you can set and achieve new goals year after year:

- **Break Long-Term Goals into Short-Term Milestones**: Long-term goals are great for vision and motivation, but they can also feel overwhelming. To make them achievable, break them down into smaller, incremental milestones. For example, if your long-term goal is to bench press 150kg, break it down into monthly or quarterly targets (e.g., adding 5kg every month).

- **Set Performance and Process Goals**: Performance goals are outcome-based (e.g., hitting a new personal best), but process goals focus on improving the techniques, habits, and strategies that lead to performance success. For example, your performance goal might be to increase your 1-rep max in the military press, while your process goal could be improving your form, consistency in training, or nutrition habits.

- **Challenge Yourself with New Lifts and Variations**: In addition to improving your core lifts (bench press, military press, and bent-over rows), challenge yourself by adding new exercises or variations to your routine. These could include movements like incline bench press, overhead squats, or Romanian deadlifts. By diversifying your training, you keep things interesting and target muscles from different angles, enhancing overall strength development.

- **Celebrate Milestones and Reflect**: Celebrating milestones, no matter how small, is essential for maintaining motivation. Take the time to acknowledge your progress and reflect on how far you've come. At the same time, review your approach to see what worked and what didn't. Constant reflection is a powerful tool for fine-tuning your strategy and ensuring that you're always moving in the right direction.

4. Conclusion

Tracking your progress and adjusting your training routine is an ongoing process that evolves with your strength development. By consistently monitoring your lifts, reassessing your goals, and incorporating new training strategies, you ensure that your progress continues year after year. Remember, long-term success in strength training comes from being adaptable, patient, and willing to push through challenges. Whether you're a beginner just starting your journey or an experienced lifter striving for new heights, tracking your progress and adjusting your routine is the key to unlocking your full strength potential.

As you move forward, embrace the idea that success is not just about lifting more weight—it's about constantly improving, learning from setbacks, and setting your sights on new challenges. Strength mastery is a lifelong pursuit, and by applying the principles outlined in this book, you will be well on your way to achieving your goals and surpassing them, time and time again.

Chapter 1: The Science of Strength Training

Strength training is more than just lifting weights; it's a systematic approach to enhancing the body's power, resilience, and functionality. Whether you're looking to improve athletic performance, increase muscle mass, or simply become stronger in daily life, understanding the science behind strength training is crucial for achieving long-term success. This chapter will delve into the physiological and biomechanical principles that drive strength gains, how progressive overload works, and why recovery and nutrition are indispensable components of any strength-building program.

Understanding Muscle Physiology and Biomechanics

At its core, strength training focuses on the development of muscle fibers through resistance. When you lift weights or perform other forms of resistance exercise, the muscles experience microtears, which then repair and grow back stronger. This process is known as **muscle hypertrophy**. To understand how this works, it's helpful to break down the key elements involved in muscle physiology:

- **Muscle Fibers**: Human muscles are made up of two main types of fibers: Type I (slow-twitch) and Type II (fast-twitch). Type I fibers are more endurance-oriented and are used for lighter, repetitive movements, while Type II fibers are larger and more powerful, recruited during intense, explosive efforts like heavy lifting. Strength training predominantly targets Type II fibers, which grow larger in response to heavy load and high-intensity training.
- **Muscle Contraction**: When lifting weights, the muscles contract as a result of signals from the brain. This contraction happens through the interaction of actin and myosin filaments within muscle cells. The more forcefully these filaments interact, the greater the contraction—and ultimately the stronger the muscle. Training with progressively heavier loads stimulates the muscle fibers to adapt, creating a stronger, more efficient muscle.
- **Biomechanics**: The science of movement, or biomechanics, plays a critical role in strength training. Understanding the optimal angles, joint mechanics, and body positioning during lifts ensures maximum force production while minimizing injury risk. Proper alignment and efficient movement patterns ensure that the targeted muscles are activated, and unnecessary stress is not placed on the joints.

For example, when performing a **bench press**, the shoulder blades should be retracted and depressed to create a stable base for pressing the barbell. This minimizes stress on the shoulder joints and maximizes power generation through the chest, shoulders, and triceps.

Progressive Overload Principles

Progressive overload is the cornerstone of any strength training program. This principle dictates that in order to continue making strength gains, you must gradually increase the intensity of your workouts. Without progressive overload, your body will adapt to the same stress levels, and progress will plateau. There are several ways to apply this principle:

1. **Increase Weight**: The most straightforward way to progressively overload is by increasing the amount of weight you lift. If you bench press 135 pounds for 8 reps today, your goal might be to lift 145 pounds for the same number of reps next week. Gradually adding more weight forces your muscles to handle greater stress, resulting in growth.

2. **Increase Reps or Sets**: Another form of progressive overload involves increasing the number of repetitions or sets you perform at a given weight. If you bench press 135 pounds for 8 reps today, try for 10 reps the next time. The additional volume stresses the muscle fibers further, leading to growth.

3. **Increase Training Frequency**: By training a particular muscle group more frequently, you can push your body to adapt quicker. For example, if you're training chest once per week, you might try training it twice a week, focusing on different variations of the bench press to target different aspects of the chest.

4. **Manipulate Tempo**: Slowing down the tempo (the speed at which you lift and lower the weight) increases the time under tension, which can enhance strength gains. Performing a bench press with a 3-second descent and a 1-second ascent increases muscle fatigue, leading to hypertrophy.

5. **Focus on Form and Execution**: Another critical aspect of progressive overload is improving the quality of your lifts. Each time you perfect your technique—whether it's a more controlled movement or ensuring full range of motion—you are effectively increasing the intensity, even without changing the weight.

No matter which method you use, the key is to make incremental changes. Small, consistent progress is much more sustainable in the long term than trying to make huge leaps all at once. The body responds well to gradual increases in intensity, which is why programs based on progressive overload often yield the best results.

The Role of Nutrition and Recovery in Strength Building

While exercise is the stimulus for muscle growth, **nutrition** and **recovery** are what enable muscle adaptation and growth to actually take place.

Nutrition

Carbohydrates are the body's primary energy source during high-intensity training. Consuming enough carbs ensures that the muscles have enough glycogen (stored energy) for your lifts. Healthy fats are essential for hormone production, including testosterone, which plays a significant role in muscle growth.

Hydration is equally important. Dehydration can hinder performance, decrease strength output, and increase the risk of injury. Be sure to drink enough water throughout the day to maintain peak performance.

Recovery

In addition to sleep, **active recovery** such as light stretching, foam rolling, and mobility exercises can improve circulation and reduce muscle soreness. It's essential to strike a balance between hard training and sufficient rest to prevent overtraining, which can lead to burnout and injury.

The Importance of Mastering Foundational Lifts

While strength training encompasses a wide variety of exercises, the **bench press**, **military press**, and **bent-over row** are foundational lifts that recruit multiple muscle groups and build total-body strength. Mastering these three exercises forms the basis for a well-rounded strength program.

The bench press primarily targets the chest, shoulders, and triceps. The military press emphasizes the shoulders, triceps, and upper chest, while the bent-over row focuses on the back, particularly the lats, traps, and rhomboids. Each of these movements, when executed correctly, engages the core and stabilizing muscles, providing a functional strength base that improves overall athleticism and enhances performance in everyday activities.

By mastering these lifts, you can develop raw strength and enhance functional power, which transfers to a wide range of other exercises and physical activities. Furthermore, because these lifts are compound movements, they also allow for significant load progression, making them ideal for continued muscle growth and strength.

Setting Goals and Tracking Progress

The key to success in strength training, as with any endeavor, is goal setting. Without clear objectives, it's easy to lose motivation or veer off track. Start by setting both **short-term** and **long-term** goals. A short-term goal might be to add 5 pounds to your bench press in the next month, while a long-term goal could be to bench press twice your body weight within the next year.

Tracking progress is just as essential as setting goals. Documenting the weights you lift, the number of sets and reps, and any changes in technique helps to provide measurable data on your progress. Apps or training journals are useful tools for tracking performance and ensuring that you're consistently pushing yourself to improve.

Remember that progress is not always linear. You will encounter plateaus and setbacks, but with patience and consistency, strength gains will come. The key is to stay focused on the process, adjust when necessary, and always look for ways to improve.

Conclusion

In this chapter, we've covered the foundational principles behind strength training, focusing on muscle physiology, progressive overload, and the importance of recovery and nutrition. Mastering the bench press, military press, and bent-over rows relies on understanding these core principles, as they provide the basis for achieving maximum strength. By integrating these scientific principles into your training program, you set yourself up for success and lasting gains. In the next chapter, we will explore the equipment needed to perform these exercises safely and effectively.

Chapter 2: Equipment 101

In the world of strength training, the right equipment can make all the difference between achieving optimal results and risking injury. Whether you're working out at a gym or setting up your home gym, understanding the essential equipment used for foundational lifts like the **bench press**, **military press**, and **bent-over rows** is crucial to ensure safety, efficiency, and progression. This chapter will cover the different types of equipment needed for these exercises, how to properly set them up for safe and effective lifts, and how to choose the right weights to match your strength level and training goals.

The Bench Press Apparatus

The **bench press** is one of the most iconic strength training exercises, known for building upper body power. It requires a bench and a barbell, but several considerations need to be made to ensure that you're lifting safely and effectively.

- **Flat Bench**: The flat bench is the standard for bench pressing. It provides a stable surface for you to lie on while pressing the barbell up and down. It's essential that the bench is sturdy and well-constructed to handle heavy loads without wobbling. Look for benches with adjustable heights or incline settings if you plan to experiment with different angles, such as incline or decline bench presses.
- **Barbell**: The **barbell** is the main tool used in the bench press. Standard barbells typically weigh 20 kg (44 lbs), though variations exist for lighter or heavier lifting. The barbell should have knurling (textured grips) on the shaft to provide a secure grip for your hands, especially when lifting heavy. Be sure that the barbell you use is in good condition and free from rust or damage.
- **Weight Plates**: To load the barbell with the desired resistance, you will need weight plates. These can come in a variety of materials, from rubber-coated to steel, and they typically range from 1.25 kg (2.5 lbs) to 45 kg (100 lbs). Select plates that fit securely on the barbell and ensure that they are evenly distributed to maintain balance.
- **Collars/Clamps**: These are used to secure the weight plates onto the barbell. While it's easy to overlook, collars are vital for safety, especially when using heavy weights. Without them, the plates could shift or even slide off, leading to accidents. Ensure your collars are tight enough to hold the plates in place without moving during the lift.

- **Power Rack (Optional)**: A **power rack** is highly recommended for bench pressing, especially when lifting heavy loads. It allows you to perform the exercise safely without a spotter. The rack should have adjustable safety bars set at a height where the barbell will rest if you fail the lift. This feature is crucial for avoiding injuries, as it provides a safety net in case you cannot complete the rep.

The Military Press Setup

The **military press** (also known as the overhead press) is a classic exercise for building shoulder strength and stability. The setup is slightly different from the bench press, as it requires overhead motion, but the equipment used is similar.

- **Barbell and Weight Plates**: Just like the bench press, the military press requires a barbell and weight plates. In most cases, you can use the same barbell you would for the bench press, as long as it is loaded with the appropriate weight for your training goals.
- **Rack or Squat Rack**: Unlike the bench press, the military press begins from a standing position with the barbell lifted to shoulder height. The **squat rack** or **power rack** is used to elevate the barbell at a height that allows you to lift it into position. Make sure the rack is sturdy and that the bar is set at the correct height for your body. It's important that the bar is at chest or shoulder level so that you can lift it safely without straining your back or shoulders.
- **Adjustable Bench (Optional)**: While not essential, an **adjustable bench** can be used to add an incline or decline angle to your press, shifting the emphasis slightly onto different parts of the shoulder or upper chest. It's crucial that any bench you use for the military press is stable and securely locked into place.
- **Spotter**: In some cases, a spotter may be necessary, particularly when lifting heavy overhead. A good spotter will be able to assist you if you encounter difficulty with a lift, helping to avoid any risk of dropping the barbell onto your head or shoulders.

The Bent-Over Row Setup

The **bent-over row** is a pulling exercise designed to strengthen the back, shoulders, and arms. It's typically performed using a barbell, dumbbells, or machines, but the setup for free-weight bent-over rows requires specific attention to form and safety.

- **Barbell or Dumbbells**: For the **barbell bent-over row**, the setup is very similar to that of the bench press or military press. The barbell should be loaded with the appropriate weight, and you should stand with your feet hip-width apart to maintain balance while pulling. The **dumbbell bent-over row** allows for a more unilateral approach, where you lift each arm individually, which can help correct muscle imbalances.
- **Weight Plates**: Similar to the bench press, the bent-over row uses weight plates to load the barbell. It's important that the plates are securely fastened with collars to prevent them from sliding off as you pull.
- **Platform or Weight Bench (Optional)**: While the bent-over row can be done from the floor, using a weight bench or a platform for support can provide a more controlled range of motion and reduce strain on your lower back. In a standing row, maintain a slight bend at the knees and focus on hinging at the hips, keeping your chest high and back straight to protect your spine.
- **T-Bar Row (Optional)**: For a variation of the bent-over row, the **T-bar row** is often used to isolate the back muscles with a different grip and angle. This variation requires a T-bar machine or a landmine attachment, which can provide a different type of resistance.

Proper Form and Setup for Safety

Setting up for any exercise is just as important as performing the movement itself. Proper form is critical not only for maximizing performance but also for preventing injury.

- **Bench Press Setup**: To set up for the bench press, lie flat on the bench with your feet planted firmly on the floor. Your eyes should be directly under the bar. Grip the bar slightly wider than shoulder-width, ensuring your wrists are straight and aligned with your elbows. Lower the bar slowly to your chest, maintaining control, and press it back up to the starting position. Engage your core throughout the movement, and avoid letting your feet leave the floor or arching your back excessively.

- **Military Press Setup**: Before you begin the military press, stand with the barbell positioned at shoulder height, either in a squat rack or by lifting it off the floor. Grip the barbell just outside shoulder-width with your elbows slightly in front of the bar. Engage your core and press the bar overhead in a straight line, keeping your body in a stable, upright position. Avoid leaning back or overextending your lower back, which can lead to injury.

- **Bent-Over Row Setup**: To perform the bent-over row, stand with your feet shoulder-width apart and hinge at the hips, keeping your back flat and chest up. Grip the barbell with a pronated (overhand) grip and pull the barbell towards your lower chest or upper abdomen, ensuring that your elbows stay close to your body. Keep your core engaged throughout the movement to protect your spine from excessive strain.

Choosing the Right Weights and Adjusting for Progress

Selecting the right weights for each exercise is crucial to ensure you are challenging your muscles without overloading them, which can lead to injury.

- **Starting Light**: If you're new to strength training or a particular exercise, it's important to start light. Mastering the technique should be your primary focus before adding weight. Lifting too heavy too soon can compromise your form and increase the risk of injury.
- **Progressing Gradually**: As you gain strength, you can gradually increase the weight. Aim for a weight that allows you to perform the exercise with good form while still being challenging. For compound exercises like the bench press and military press, aim for sets of 6-12 reps, which is a range that promotes both strength and hypertrophy.
- **Adjusting for Plateaus**: If you hit a plateau and aren't making progress, it may be time to adjust the weights or use progressive techniques like tempo manipulation or incorporating accessory movements to strengthen weak points.

Conclusion

The right equipment, proper setup, and correct form are the cornerstones of a successful strength training program. By understanding how to use the bench press, military press, and bent-over row apparatus safely and effectively, you're setting yourself up for success in building total-body strength. As you progress, remember that selecting the appropriate weights and maintaining safety should always be your priority. In the next chapter, we will explore the core movements of these exercises and how they fit into a well-rounded strength training regimen.

Chapter 3: Understanding the Core Movements

In strength training, the **bench press**, **military press**, and **bent-over rows** are three of the most effective compound exercises for building upper-body strength and overall athletic performance. These foundational lifts are integral to a full-body workout because they target multiple muscle groups simultaneously, engage stabilizing muscles, and promote functional strength. This chapter will explore how these core movements fit into a complete training regimen, the muscles they target, and the importance of complementary accessory exercises to enhance your strength and prevent imbalances.

The Bench Press: Targeting the Chest, Shoulders, and Triceps

The **bench press** is widely regarded as the gold standard for building upper body pushing strength. Its main muscles targeted are the **pectoralis major** (chest), **deltoids** (shoulders), and **triceps brachii** (arms). However, the bench press also engages a range of secondary muscles that contribute to stability and control.

Primary Muscles

- **Pectoralis Major**: The chest muscles are the prime movers in the bench press, especially the sternal part of the pectoralis major. The wider the grip, the more the chest is emphasized.
- **Deltoids (Shoulders)**: The anterior deltoids (front part of the shoulders) work to stabilize the bar and assist with the press.
- **Triceps**: The triceps play a crucial role in locking out the bar at the top of the movement and are heavily involved during the final portion of the press.

Secondary Muscles

- **Serratus Anterior**: The muscles on the sides of the rib cage help with the stabilization of the scapulae, especially during the lowering phase of the lift.
- **Rhomboids and Trapezius**: These upper back muscles stabilize the shoulder blades, keeping them retracted and preventing shoulder injury.
- **Core**: A strong core is essential for maintaining proper body position on the bench, especially when lifting heavy.

How it fits into a full-body workout:

The bench press is a **compound exercise**, meaning it works several large muscle groups at once. It can be performed on a dedicated upper-body day or integrated into a full-body workout routine. The bench press complements other pressing movements, such as the **military press**, and pulling exercises like the **bent-over row**, balancing push-pull dynamics for optimal strength development.

The Military Press: Strengthening Shoulders and Triceps

The **military press** (or overhead press) is a fundamental overhead pressing movement that strengthens the shoulders, upper chest, and triceps, while also engaging the core and stabilizer muscles.

Primary Muscles

- **Deltoids**: The military press targets all three heads of the deltoids, with a particular emphasis on the anterior and medial (front and middle) deltoid muscles.
- **Triceps**: The triceps assist with the pressing motion and help extend the elbows, especially as the bar is locked overhead.
- **Upper Chest**: The upper portion of the pectoralis major is involved in the lift, especially when pressing at slightly forward angles.

Secondary Muscles

- **Upper Back**: The trapezius and rhomboids stabilize the shoulders and neck region, ensuring control during the lift.
- **Core**: The core muscles (rectus abdominis, obliques, and lower back) must engage to maintain stability and prevent excessive lower back arching, particularly when the weight is heavy.
- **Forearms and Grip**: Grip strength and forearm stability are essential for controlling the barbell overhead.

How it fits into a full-body workout:

The military press can be performed as a standalone lift on shoulder or upper-body days. It works synergistically with other pressing movements, like the bench press, and pulling movements, such as the bent-over row, to create a well-rounded upper-body workout. The vertical press pattern of the military press contrasts with the horizontal push of the bench press, offering variety for shoulder development and functional strength.

The Bent-Over Row: Building the Back and Strengthening the Posterior Chain

The **bent-over row** is a classic pulling exercise that targets the **posterior chain** (the muscles along the back of the body), including the lats, rhomboids, traps, and lower back. It is a key exercise for building strength and mass in the back, balancing out the pushing movements of the bench press and military press.

Primary Muscles

- **Latissimus Dorsi**: The lats are the main muscles worked in the bent-over row, responsible for pulling the arms downward and inward. They are essential for creating a V-shaped back.
- **Rhomboids**: Located between the shoulder blades, the rhomboids retract the scapulae, pulling them toward the spine. This helps with shoulder stability and posture.
- **Trapezius**: The traps assist in scapular retraction and shoulder stability. The middle and lower parts of the traps are engaged when pulling the barbell toward the torso.

Secondary Muscles

- **Biceps**: While the biceps are secondary muscles in the bent-over row, they assist with elbow flexion and control the bar as you pull.
- **Posterior Deltoids**: The rear delts help stabilize the shoulders during the row and assist in the movement, especially when pulling with heavier loads.
- **Core**: Like the military press, the core plays a significant role in stabilizing the body and maintaining a neutral spine throughout the row. Proper engagement of the abs and lower back is critical to prevent injury.

How it fits into a full-body workout:

The bent-over row is an excellent pulling exercise that should be incorporated into any upper-body workout, especially on back or pulling-focused days. It balances out the pushing exercises, ensuring that both the anterior and posterior parts of the upper body are trained effectively. Incorporating rows into your routine enhances upper back strength, posture, and scapular mobility, making it a vital exercise for functional movement.

The Importance of Accessory Exercises

While the bench press, military press, and bent-over row form the core of a strength program, **accessory exercises** are equally important for addressing muscle imbalances, strengthening weak points, and improving overall movement patterns.

For the Bench Press

- **Tricep Dips**: Dips are a great accessory movement to strengthen the triceps, helping with the lockout phase of the bench press.
- **Rotator Cuff Exercises**: Strengthening the rotator cuff muscles is crucial for shoulder health and injury prevention. External rotations and band pull-aparts are effective exercises.
- **Chest Flys**: These isolate the chest muscles and can help develop more muscle mass in the pectorals, complementing the press.

For the Military Press

- **Lateral Raises**: These target the middle deltoid and can help balance out shoulder development for improved pressing strength.
- **Face Pulls**: This exercise targets the rear deltoids and upper traps, enhancing shoulder stability and posture.
- **Shrugs**: Shrugging helps build trap strength, which contributes to shoulder stability during the press.

For the Bent-Over Row

- **Pull-Ups/Chin-Ups**: These are excellent bodyweight exercises for developing the back muscles, particularly the lats and biceps.
- **Single-Arm Dumbbell Rows**: This exercise isolates each side of the back and helps correct muscle imbalances.
- **Back Extensions**: Strengthening the lower back is crucial for maintaining proper posture and spinal alignment during rowing movements.

Integrating the Core Movements into a Full-Body Workout Routine

When building a full-body workout, it's essential to strategically integrate these core lifts with accessory exercises for a balanced approach. A typical weekly strength training program may look like this:

Day 1 (Upper Body Push/Pull)

- Bench Press (4 sets of 6-8 reps)
- Military Press (3 sets of 6-8 reps)
- Bent-Over Rows (4 sets of 6-8 reps)
- Accessory: Tricep Dips, Pull-Ups

Day 2 (Lower Body/Core)

- Squats, Deadlifts, Lunges
- Core Work (Planks, Leg Raises)

Day 3 (Upper Body Push/Pull)

- Bench Press (4 sets of 6-8 reps)
- Military Press (3 sets of 6-8 reps)
- Accessory: Lateral Raises, Face Pulls, Shrugs

Day 4 (Active Recovery)

Mobility Work, Stretching, Light Cardio

Conclusion

Understanding how the bench press, military press, and bent-over row fit into a full-body workout is key to structuring an effective and balanced strength training routine. These compound exercises target large muscle groups and work synergistically to promote total-body strength and functional fitness. Complementing them with accessory movements ensures that you develop all the muscles needed for powerful and injury-free performance. In the next chapter, we will dive deeper into common mistakes and how to avoid them, so you can perfect your form and continue to progress safely and effectively.

Chapter 4: Common Mistakes and How to Avoid Them

In any strength training journey, understanding the correct technique for the bench press, military press, and bent-over row is crucial for long-term progress and injury prevention. Despite their effectiveness, these exercises are often performed incorrectly, leading to suboptimal results or, worse, injuries. This chapter will explore the most common mistakes made during these three foundational lifts and provide corrective techniques to enhance performance, prevent injury, and ensure consistent gains. Whether you're a beginner or an experienced lifter, mastering form is the key to maximizing strength.

Common Mistakes in the Bench Press

The bench press is one of the most widely performed exercises, but it's also one of the most prone to mistakes. Here are the key errors often seen in the bench press and how to correct them:

Incorrect Bar Path

- **Mistake**: Letting the bar drift forward or down towards the neck rather than following a straight line.
- **Correction**: The bar should travel in a slightly diagonal path, coming down to your mid-chest. This helps ensure maximum chest activation and reduces strain on the shoulders.

Feet Off the Floor

- **Mistake**: Lifting your feet off the floor or placing them on the bench.
- **Correction**: Keep your feet planted firmly on the floor to provide stability and activate your legs. This creates a solid base for generating force and maintaining body alignment.

Elbows Flaring Out Too Much

- **Mistake**: Letting your elbows flare out at a 90-degree angle from your body.
- **Correction**: Aim to keep your elbows at about a 45-degree angle to your torso. This will keep the shoulders in a safer position and improve pressing power.

Lifting Your Hips Off the Bench

- **Mistake**: Arching your lower back too excessively, leading to the hips lifting off the bench.
- **Correction**: Maintain a neutral spine throughout the lift, ensuring that only your chest and feet are in contact with the bench. A slight arch in the lower back is fine, but avoid excessive lumbar extension.

Not Engaging the Lats

- **Mistake**: Failing to activate the lats during the lowering phase of the bench press.
- **Correction**: Before you press, engage your lats by squeezing them down and back. This helps with stability, keeps your shoulders protected, and improves overall pressing power.

Bouncing the Bar Off the Chest

- **Mistake**: Letting the bar bounce off the chest in an effort to use momentum for the lift.
- **Correction**: Lower the bar under control and pause for a brief moment before pressing it back up. This ensures full muscle activation and minimizes the risk of injury.

Common Mistakes in the Military Press

The military press is an essential lift for shoulder and upper body development, but it requires precision to execute correctly. Common errors include:

Overarching the Lower Back

- **Mistake**: Using excessive lower back arching to press the bar overhead, which can strain the spine.
- **Correction**: Engage your core and squeeze your glutes to prevent arching. Maintain a neutral spine throughout the press to protect your lower back.

Elbows Flaring Too Much

- **Mistake**: Flailing the elbows out excessively during the press.
- **Correction**: Keep the elbows slightly in front of the bar to minimize shoulder strain. The bar should follow a vertical path rather than a forward arc.

Pressing Too Far Behind the Head

- **Mistake**: Pressing the bar too far behind the head, often resulting in shoulder discomfort.
- **Correction**: Press the bar directly overhead, staying in line with the ears. This helps keep the shoulder joints in a safer, more stable position.

Not Engaging the Core

- **Mistake**: Failing to engage the core, which leads to instability and poor posture.
- **Correction**: Brace your core tightly before initiating the press. This provides support for your spine and helps maintain a stable torso throughout the movement.

Relying Too Much on the Legs

- **Mistake**: Using excessive leg drive to assist with the press, turning the movement into a push press.
- **Correction**: The military press should be performed with minimal leg involvement. Only engage the legs if you're performing a push press or jerk variation. Focus on pressing with the shoulders and arms.

Common Mistakes in the Bent-Over Row

The bent-over row is an excellent pulling movement, but it can lead to imbalances or back issues if not performed correctly. Here are common errors and how to fix them:

Rounded Back

- **Mistake**: Allowing the back to round during the rowing motion, which places undue stress on the spine and increases the risk of injury.
- **Correction**: Maintain a neutral spine by engaging your core and pulling your shoulder blades back. A slight bend in the knees is acceptable, but the back should stay straight throughout the movement.

Using Too Much Weight

- **Mistake**: Lifting a weight that's too heavy, resulting in a lack of control and improper form.
- **Correction**: Choose a weight that allows you to control the movement with a full range of motion. Focus on controlled movements rather than attempting to lift as much as possible.

Not Retracting the Scapula

- **Mistake**: Failing to engage the upper back by not retracting the shoulder blades during the row.
- **Correction**: Initiate the movement by pulling the shoulder blades back and down before bending your elbows. This engages the upper back muscles more effectively and protects the shoulders.

Pulling the Elbows Too High

- **Mistake**: Lifting the elbows too high, which shifts the focus to the traps and reduces activation of the lats.
- **Correction**: Keep the elbows at a 45-degree angle to your torso, aiming to keep them close to the body as you row. This engages the lats more effectively.

Jerking or Using Momentum

- **Mistake**: Using momentum to swing the weight rather than engaging the muscles in a controlled fashion.
- **Correction**: Perform the movement slowly and deliberately, ensuring each rep is controlled. Focus on squeezing the muscles at the top of the movement before lowering the weight.

Preventing Injuries and Long-Term Issues

Mastering proper technique not only improves strength but also plays a critical role in preventing injury. Here are some general tips to safeguard your body during strength training:

1. **Warm-Up Properly**: Always perform a dynamic warm-up before lifting to prepare your muscles, joints, and nervous system for the work ahead. Focus on the muscle groups you'll be training and include mobility exercises for the shoulders, hips, and back.

2. **Use Full Range of Motion**: Avoid cutting the range of motion short, which can lead to muscular imbalances. For example, in the bench press, ensure that the bar touches your chest each time, and in rows, aim for a full retraction of the scapula.

3. **Progress Gradually**: Progressive overload is crucial, but adding weight too quickly can cause injuries. Increase weight by small increments and focus on maintaining form rather than lifting heavy weight prematurely.

4. **Listen to Your Body**: Pay attention to any discomfort or pain. It's normal to feel muscle fatigue, but sharp or persistent pain can be a sign of overuse or poor form. Always back off if you feel something isn't right.

5. **Prioritize Recovery**: Strength training puts significant stress on your muscles and joints, so recovery is just as important as the lifting itself. Ensure you're getting enough rest, proper nutrition, and stretching to maintain flexibility and muscle health.

Conclusion

Avoiding common mistakes in the bench press, military press, and bent-over row is crucial for building strength, improving performance, and preventing injury. By focusing on proper form, listening to your body, and implementing corrective techniques, you'll be able to progress efficiently and safely in your strength training journey. In the next chapter, we'll explore how to structure your workout program to maximize results and incorporate these movements for long-term success.

Chapter 5: How to Structure Your Program

Designing a strength training program is an essential step in your journey toward mastery of the bench press, military press, and bent-over rows. Whether you're a beginner or an advanced lifter, structuring a program effectively will ensure that you develop strength, enhance performance, and avoid plateaus. This chapter provides a guide for creating a balanced workout plan that aligns with your goals, fitness level, and desired outcomes.

Designing a Balanced Workout Plan

A well-structured strength training program focuses on progressively increasing load and intensity while maintaining balance across muscle groups. Here's how to design a program that will effectively target all the muscles involved in the bench press, military press, and bent-over row:

Establish Your Goals

- **Strength Focus**: If your goal is to maximize strength, prioritize compound movements (bench press, military press, and bent-over rows) with low-to-moderate reps (3-6 per set) and high intensity. Focus on lifting progressively heavier weights while maintaining proper form.
- **Hypertrophy Focus**: If muscle growth is the goal, work in the 6-12 rep range with moderate to heavy weights. Incorporate accessory exercises and increase volume to target muscle fatigue and stimulate muscle growth.
- **Endurance Focus**: If endurance is your goal, aim for higher reps (12-20 per set) with lighter weights, incorporating techniques like supersets or circuit training to improve muscular stamina.

Program Frequency

Beginners

- Day 1: Bench press, military press, accessory shoulder and chest exercises.
- Day 2: Bent-over row, accessory back and arm exercises.
- Day 3: Compound lifts (lower body or full body with moderate-intensity variations).

- **Intermediate Lifters**: Aim for 4-5 training days per week. A typical program may include a push-pull split (e.g., upper body push/upper body pull/lower body) to allow sufficient recovery while increasing training volume and intensity.
- **Advanced Lifters**: 5-6 days per week, incorporating specialized programs like push-pull-legs, or periodized programs that cycle intensity and volume across weeks to maximize strength and hypertrophy.

Volume and Intensity

- **Strength Focus**: Use lower volume but high intensity. This means fewer sets (3-5 sets) with low reps (3-6 reps) at higher intensities (80-90% of your 1RM).
- **Hypertrophy Focus**: Moderate intensity and volume. Perform 4-6 sets of 6-12 reps, working with weights that are around 70-80% of your 1RM.
- **Endurance Focus**: High volume, moderate-to-low intensity. Aim for 3-5 sets of 12-20 reps with lighter weights (50-70% of your 1RM).

Progressive Overload

- **Increase Weight**: Gradually increase the weight lifted each week or every other week.
- **Increase Reps or Sets**: Start with a moderate weight and gradually increase the number of reps or sets you perform.
- **Adjust Tempo**: Slow down the eccentric (lowering) phase of the lift to increase time under tension, or use a pause at the bottom of the lift to build strength and stability.

Combining Compound and Isolation Exercises

While the bench press, military press, and bent-over rows are essential compound lifts that target multiple muscle groups, accessory exercises can complement them by focusing on specific muscles, preventing imbalances, and improving your performance. Here's how to structure your program:

Primary Compound Movements

- **Bench Press**: Target chest, shoulders, and triceps.
- **Military Press**: Focus on shoulders, triceps, and upper chest.
- **Bent-Over Row**: Target the back, traps, biceps, and rear delts.

Accessory Movements

- **Chest and Shoulders**: Dumbbell presses, chest flyes, lateral raises, front raises.
- **Back and Biceps**: Lat pulldowns, dumbbell rows, barbell curls, face pulls.
- **Triceps and Forearms**: Tricep dips, tricep pushdowns, wrist curls.

3. These exercises not only help build muscle and increase strength but also protect the joints and tendons involved in the primary lifts, reducing the risk of injury and overuse.

4. **Core Training**

    A strong core is vital for stability and posture during all strength movements. Incorporate core exercises like planks, Russian twists, leg raises, and cable woodchoppers to build functional strength and improve overall lifting technique.

Frequency, Volume, and Intensity Recommendations

The frequency, volume, and intensity of your program will vary based on your level and goals. Here's how to apply these principles to different stages of lifting:

For Beginners

- **Frequency**: 3-4 days per week.
- **Volume**: Moderate (3-4 sets per exercise, 8-12 reps).
- **Intensity**: Moderate (50-70% of 1RM).
- **Program Structure**: Full-body workouts, focusing on basic form and building endurance.

For Intermediate Lifters

- **Frequency**: 4-5 days per week.
- **Volume**: Higher (4-6 sets per exercise, 6-10 reps).
- **Intensity**: Moderate to heavy (70-85% of 1RM).
- **Program Structure**: Split programs like push/pull/legs, with accessory exercises to target weak points.

For Advanced Lifters

- **Frequency**: 5-6 days per week.
- **Volume**: Very high (4-8 sets per exercise, 3-6 reps for strength, 6-12 reps for hypertrophy).
- **Intensity**: Heavy (85-95% of 1RM).
- **Program Structure**: Periodized programs with varying intensity and volume, along with advanced techniques like supersets, drop sets, and training to failure.

Tracking Progress

Tracking your progress is essential to measure improvements and make necessary adjustments to your training program. Use the following strategies to stay on top of your strength gains:

1. **Log Your Lifts**: Keep a workout journal or use an app to track the weights, sets, and reps for each exercise. This will help you see when it's time to increase the load or change your program.
2. **Assess Strength Gains**: Track improvements in key lifts (bench press, military press, and bent-over rows). Periodically test your 1RM to measure overall progress.
3. **Monitor Recovery**: Record how well you recover after each workout. If you're consistently feeling fatigued or noticing declining performance, it may be time to adjust your intensity or recovery strategies.
4. **Set Milestones**: Break down larger goals into smaller, manageable milestones. For example, instead of aiming for a 100-pound bench press increase, set smaller incremental goals like increasing your 5-rep max by 5 pounds each month.

Conclusion

A well-structured program is the foundation of your strength training journey. By combining the bench press, military press, and bent-over rows with accessory exercises, managing frequency, volume, and intensity, and tracking your progress, you'll be on the path to strength mastery. In the following chapters, we'll dive deeper into each of these lifts, providing specific techniques, variations, and strategies to help you reach new levels of power and performance.

Chapter 6: The Bench Press: Overview and Benefits

The bench press is often considered the cornerstone of upper body strength training. This classic lift has earned its place as a fundamental exercise in powerlifting, bodybuilding, and general strength programs. In this chapter, we'll delve into the anatomy of the bench press, explore its benefits, and discuss how mastering this movement can lead to impressive gains in both strength and muscle development.

Anatomy of the Bench Press

The bench press is a compound movement, meaning it recruits multiple muscle groups simultaneously. Its primary muscles involved are:

1. **Pectoralis Major**: The chest muscles are the main drivers during the press. The bench press effectively targets the clavicular (upper) and sternal (middle and lower) portions of the chest, making it a powerful exercise for overall chest development.
2. **Deltoids**: The shoulders, particularly the anterior (front) deltoids, assist in pressing the barbell away from the chest. They stabilize the movement and help initiate the press, contributing to overall shoulder strength.
3. **Triceps Brachii**: The triceps play a crucial role in locking out the elbows at the top of the press. As you push the bar upward, the triceps work to extend your arms, contributing to the power needed for the lift.
4. **Rhomboids and Trapezius**: While the rhomboids and traps aren't the primary movers, they provide stabilization through the scapular retraction process, helping ensure a strong and safe press.
5. **Serratus Anterior**: This muscle, which helps protract the scapula, assists in the movement by keeping the shoulder blade stable and supporting the pressing motion.

Understanding these key muscle groups helps explain why the bench press is such an effective exercise for building upper body strength. By engaging both large and small muscle groups, it maximizes overall muscular development while improving functional strength.

Key Benefits of the Bench Press

The bench press offers numerous benefits that extend beyond mere aesthetic improvement:

1. **Upper Body Strength**: One of the most obvious benefits is the increase in upper body strength. A stronger bench press translates into better performance in other lifts and daily activities, as well as increased force production for athletes involved in contact sports or explosive movements.

2. **Muscle Hypertrophy**: The bench press is an essential exercise for building chest, shoulder, and tricep size. Consistently challenging these muscle groups with progressive overload leads to hypertrophy (muscle growth) and improved muscular endurance.

3. **Functional Strength**: The motion of the bench press mimics various real-world movements, such as pushing, pressing, or lifting heavy objects. As such, mastering the bench press builds functional strength that translates into better performance in sports and physical tasks.

4. **Bone Density and Joint Health**: Regularly performing the bench press, particularly with progressive loading, can help increase bone density, particularly in the wrists, elbows, and shoulders. Additionally, the controlled range of motion helps reinforce healthy joint movement, contributing to long-term joint integrity.

5. **Improved Confidence**: The bench press is a key strength marker for many lifters. As you increase your bench press performance, you'll likely experience a boost in self-confidence, which can spill over into other areas of life.

Variations of the Bench Press

While the traditional barbell bench press is the most well-known variation, there are several other ways to perform this exercise to target muscles from different angles and provide variety to your training routine:

1. **Incline Bench Press**: Performed on an inclined bench (usually set at a 30–45-degree angle), this variation places more emphasis on the upper chest and shoulders. It's an excellent way to develop the upper portion of the pectorals and deltoids.

2. **Decline Bench Press**: This variation is performed on a declined bench, targeting the lower chest. It can be an excellent option for individuals looking to enhance the development of the sternal portion of the pectorals.

3. **Dumbbell Bench Press**: Using dumbbells instead of a barbell allows for a greater range of motion and engages more stabilizing muscles, as each arm works independently. This variation is great for correcting imbalances and increasing overall muscle activation.

4. **Close-Grip Bench Press**: By narrowing the hand placement, this variation places more emphasis on the triceps while still working the chest and shoulders. It's a great accessory movement for improving lockout strength in the bench press.

5. **Paused Bench Press**: In this variation, you pause at the bottom of the lift for 1-2 seconds before pressing the bar back up. The pause eliminates any momentum, forcing your muscles to generate maximum force from a dead stop, which increases strength at the bottom of the lift.

6. **Floor Press**: Performed lying on the floor, this variation eliminates the leg drive and reduces the range of motion, allowing you to target the triceps and chest more effectively. It is often used to improve the upper portion of the press.

The Mental Aspect of the Bench Press

The bench press is as much a mental exercise as it is a physical one. Mental preparation and focus are essential for success in the lift. Here's how to enhance your mindset for maximal performance:

1. **Visualization**: Before you approach the bench, visualize the entire lift in your mind. Picture the bar path, your breathing, and your form. Visualizing success can boost confidence and reduce performance anxiety.

2. **Focus on Breathing**: Proper breathing is crucial for maintaining intra-abdominal pressure and stabilizing your torso. Inhale deeply as you lower the bar to your chest, and exhale forcefully as you push the bar up. Establishing a rhythmic breathing pattern helps maintain focus and energy throughout the lift.

3. **Control the Tempo**: Resist the urge to rush the lift. Lower the bar in a controlled manner, allowing your muscles to work through their full range of motion. Press the bar explosively but with control to ensure proper technique and reduce the risk of injury.

4. **Positive Self-Talk**: Use affirmations and positive self-talk to push past mental barriers. Remind yourself of your strength and past achievements. A strong mental attitude can often be the difference between hitting a PR and failing a lift.

5. **Use a Spotter**: For safety and mental confidence, always use a spotter when bench pressing heavy loads. Knowing that someone is there to assist you in case of failure allows you to push harder and take more risks in your training.

Conclusion

The bench press is a powerhouse movement that targets multiple muscle groups and delivers significant strength and hypertrophy benefits. Whether you're a beginner or an advanced lifter, mastering the bench press will not only help you build a solid upper body foundation but also contribute to greater functional strength, joint health, and mental resilience. In the next chapter, we will break down the key components of perfecting your bench press form, ensuring that you lift with precision, power, and safety.

Chapter 7: Perfecting Your Form

Form is everything when it comes to strength training, especially with foundational lifts like the bench press. A slight deviation in technique can lead to inefficiencies, prevent maximum performance, and even cause injury. In this chapter, we will break down the steps to perfect your bench press form, covering everything from hand placement to bar path, foot positioning, and breathing techniques. Mastering these details will ensure you not only perform the lift safely but also unlock your full potential.

1. Hand Placement

Your hand placement on the barbell will determine the angle of the press and which muscles are activated most. Getting this right is essential for both power and safety.

- **Standard Hand Position**: For the conventional bench press, grip the barbell with your hands slightly wider than shoulder-width apart. Your forearms should be vertical when the barbell is lowered to your chest. If your hands are too narrow or too wide, you risk compromising the efficiency of the lift, affecting your chest activation, and increasing the chance of shoulder strain.
- **Grip Type**: The most common grip is the **overhand grip**, where the palms face away from you. Ensure your thumbs are wrapped securely around the bar to prevent the bar from slipping. This grip maximizes control and power.
- **Thumb Position**: The **thumb-over grip** is the safest option. The "thumbless" or "suicide" grip (thumbs not wrapped around the bar) can increase the risk of the bar slipping, especially under heavy loads. Avoid using this grip unless you have experience and are using a spotter.
- **Elbow Angle**: When your arms are fully extended at the top of the press, your elbows should be locked out but not overextended. Keep your elbows in line with your wrists throughout the lift to prevent shoulder strain.

2. Foot Positioning

Your feet provide the base of support for the entire lift. Proper foot placement stabilizes your body, engages your core, and allows for greater power transfer.

- **Feet Flat on the Ground**: Your feet should be flat on the floor with your knees bent at about a 90-degree angle. Avoid letting your feet lift off the ground during the press as this can destabilize your body and shift focus away from the target muscles.
- **Driving Through the Heels**: While pressing, think of "driving through your heels" to activate the posterior chain (glutes, hamstrings, and lower back). This engages your core, which helps keep your body rigid and prevents arching your lower back excessively.
- **Foot Placement for Stability**: You may prefer to position your feet directly beneath your knees or slightly further out to achieve maximum stability. The key is ensuring that your feet are planted firmly to avoid any instability.
- **Leg Drive**: Some lifters use leg drive to generate power and assist the press. To do this, push your feet into the ground (without lifting your heels) as you press the bar up. This should feel like you are "bridging" your body into the bar.

3. Bar Path

The bar path refers to the trajectory that the barbell follows during the press. Maintaining a proper bar path is critical for optimizing power and reducing injury risk.

- **Lowering the Bar**: When bringing the bar down to your chest, lower it to a point just below your nipples or around the sternum area. Keep your elbows at about a 45-degree angle to your body, not flaring out excessively, which can strain the shoulders.
- **Pressing the Bar**: The bar should follow a slightly curved path. As you press the bar upward, think of pushing the bar back slightly towards your head, following a natural arc. Avoid a straight line path, as this can cause unnecessary strain on your shoulders and wrists.
- **Lockout Position**: At the top of the press, your elbows should be fully extended but not hyperextended. The bar should be directly over your shoulders, with your arms perpendicular to the floor.
- **Bar Speed**: Aim for a controlled descent and an explosive ascent. The bar should descend in a controlled manner for a few seconds (around 2-3 seconds) and then explode upward, using your full body's power. This controlled lowering phase helps in muscle recruitment and reduces the risk of injury.

4. Torso Engagement and Upper Back Positioning

Maintaining a rigid torso is essential for proper technique and power during the bench press. Many lifters neglect their upper back, which can result in a lack of stability and reduced force output.

- **Retracting the Scapula**: Before you unrack the bar, squeeze your shoulder blades together and down as if you're trying to pinch a pencil between your shoulder blades. This scapular retraction helps to stabilize your upper back and create a solid platform for pressing.
- **Chest Up**: Keeping your chest proud (lifting it slightly) is crucial for proper bench press mechanics. Imagine puffing your chest out and upward. This slight chest elevation minimizes stress on the shoulder joints and helps you press more effectively.
- **Maintaining a Neutral Spine**: Your spine should remain in a neutral position throughout the lift. This means avoiding excessive arching of your lower back, which can put undue strain on your spine and lead to injury.

5. Breathing Techniques for Maximum Efficiency

Proper breathing is critical to supporting the press and maintaining control throughout the movement.

- **Inhale Before Lowering the Bar**: Before you start lowering the bar to your chest, take a deep breath and fill your lungs with air. This helps create intra-abdominal pressure, which supports your spine and torso during the lift.
- **Brace Your Core**: As you inhale, tighten your core muscles as if you're about to get punched in the stomach. This bracing creates a solid foundation for your body, preventing any instability during the press.
- **Exhale During the Push**: As you press the bar upward, exhale forcefully. This helps you to maintain focus, reduce pressure in your chest, and push with maximum force.
- **Breathing Cadence**: Find a rhythm that works for you, but generally, aim to exhale during the concentric phase (pressing the bar up) and inhale during the eccentric phase (lowering the bar).

6. Common Mistakes to Avoid

Now that we've covered the key elements of perfect form, let's quickly review some common mistakes and how to avoid them:

- **Flared Elbows**: Allowing your elbows to flare out excessively during the descent puts unnecessary stress on the shoulder joints. Instead, aim to keep your elbows at a 45-degree angle to your body.
- **Uneven Grip**: A misaligned grip on the bar can cause uneven force distribution, leading to a lopsided press. Ensure your hands are symmetrically placed, and the bar is balanced.
- **Arching the Lower Back**: Excessive lower back arching can lead to lumbar strain. Keep your back neutral and avoid overextending your spine.
- **Bouncing the Bar**: Bouncing the bar off your chest can cause serious injuries to your ribs and sternum. Always lower the bar in a controlled manner and press it back up without relying on momentum.
- **Incomplete Lockout**: Failing to fully extend your arms at the top of the lift reduces the effectiveness of the press. Ensure you reach a complete lockout at the top.

Conclusion

Mastering the bench press form takes time and attention to detail. By focusing on hand placement, foot positioning, bar path, torso engagement, and breathing, you will ensure you are lifting with maximum power and efficiency. As with all strength training movements, consistency and patience are key to making continuous progress. In the next chapter, we will explore accessory exercises that complement the bench press, helping to strengthen weak points and prevent injury.

Chapter 8: Accessory Movements for the Bench Press

While the bench press is one of the most effective exercises for building upper body strength, it is only part of the equation when it comes to achieving true power and performance. Accessory exercises play a critical role in strengthening weak points, improving overall muscle balance, and reducing the risk of injury. In this chapter, we will explore key accessory movements designed to enhance your bench press, focusing on rotator cuff strengthening, shoulder mobility, and stabilizing muscle groups.

1. Rotator Cuff Strengthening

The rotator cuff is a group of muscles and tendons that stabilize the shoulder joint, allowing for safe and effective pressing movements. Weakness or imbalances in the rotator cuff can lead to shoulder injuries, affecting both your bench press and other upper body lifts.

- **External Rotations**: One of the best exercises to target the rotator cuff is the external rotation. Using a light dumbbell or a resistance band, hold the weight at your side and rotate your arm outward, keeping your elbow tucked in at a 90-degree angle. Perform this exercise slowly and with control to ensure you're working the smaller stabilizer muscles of the shoulder.
- **Face Pulls**: A powerful accessory exercise for the rotator cuff is the face pull, which also works the rear deltoids and upper traps. Using a rope attachment on a cable machine, set the pulley at face height and pull the rope toward your face, keeping your elbows high and squeezing your shoulder blades together. This exercise improves shoulder stability and posture, both of which are crucial for a solid bench press.
- **Prone Y Raises**: Lie face down on a bench and hold light dumbbells in each hand. With your arms extended in a "Y" shape, raise your arms overhead, squeezing your shoulder blades together. This exercise targets the lower traps and helps to improve shoulder stability, which is essential for controlling the barbell during the bench press.

- **Internal Rotations**: Although external rotations are more commonly emphasized, internal rotations can also help in balancing shoulder strength. Perform these by holding a resistance band at shoulder height and rotating your arm inward across your body. This exercise complements external rotations by targeting the internal rotator muscles, contributing to overall shoulder health.

2. Shoulder Mobility

Optimal shoulder mobility is crucial for ensuring proper bench press form and avoiding shoulder strain. Limited range of motion in the shoulders can prevent you from achieving a full range of motion during the press, reducing the effectiveness of the lift and increasing the risk of injury. Here are some exercises and stretches to enhance shoulder mobility:

- **Scapular Wall Slides**: Stand with your back against a wall, your feet a few inches away from it. Press your lower back, upper back, and head into the wall, and raise your arms into a "W" shape with your elbows bent. Slowly slide your arms up the wall, aiming for the "Y" position while maintaining contact between your arms and the wall. This exercise improves scapular mobility and engages the muscles of the rotator cuff.
- **Chest Openers**: Perform chest-opening stretches by interlacing your fingers behind your back and lifting your arms upward, squeezing your shoulder blades together. This stretch opens up the chest and enhances the flexibility needed for a proper bar path on the bench press. You can also perform this stretch using a resistance band for greater activation.
- **Shoulder Dislocations (or Pass-Throughs)**: Using a resistance band or PVC pipe, hold the object with a wide grip and slowly pass it overhead, moving the shoulders through their full range of motion. This exercise is excellent for improving shoulder flexibility and preparing the shoulders for pressing movements.

- **Band Pull-Aparts**: Hold a resistance band in front of you with both hands. Keep your arms straight and pull the band apart by retracting your shoulder blades. This exercise helps activate the posterior shoulder muscles, improving shoulder mobility and stability. It's especially useful as a warm-up before heavier bench press sets.

3. Stabilizing Muscle Groups

While the primary focus of the bench press is on the chest, shoulders, and triceps, the stability of the entire upper body contributes to your overall performance. Strengthening stabilizing muscles helps prevent compensatory movements that can limit your strength and increase your injury risk.

- **Planks**: A strong core is essential for maintaining stability during the bench press. Planks engage the abdominals, lower back, and obliques, teaching your body to maintain rigidity while pressing. Adding variations such as side planks or plank reaches can further enhance core strength and stability.

- **Dead Bugs**: The dead bug is a great exercise for improving core stability and coordination. Lie on your back with your arms extended toward the ceiling and your knees bent at 90 degrees. Slowly extend one arm and the opposite leg toward the floor while keeping your lower back pressed into the ground. Return to the starting position and alternate sides. This movement teaches control of the core, which translates to better stability while pressing heavy weights.

- **Farmer's Walks**: While this exercise primarily targets grip strength, it also works the entire body, including the core, traps, and shoulders. By holding heavy dumbbells or kettlebells in each hand, walk a set distance while maintaining an upright posture. This exercise improves your ability to stabilize your torso under load, which helps keep your body rigid during the bench press.

- **Turkish Get-Ups**: This total-body exercise improves shoulder stability, core strength, and mobility. While holding a kettlebell or dumbbell overhead, slowly move from a lying to a standing position while maintaining control of the weight. The Turkish get-up teaches stability and balance, helping you become more aware of your body's positioning during the press.

4. Triceps Strengthening

While the chest and shoulders dominate the bench press, the triceps play a key role in locking out the weight at the top of the lift. Weak triceps can limit your ability to complete the lift, especially when pressing heavy loads.

- **Triceps Dips**: Triceps dips are a great accessory movement for building triceps strength. Use parallel bars or a bench to perform the dips, lowering yourself until your upper arms are parallel to the ground. Push back up, focusing on squeezing your triceps at the top of the movement. Adding weight with a dip belt can increase the challenge as you progress.
- **Close-Grip Bench Press**: The close-grip bench press is a variation of the traditional bench press that places greater emphasis on the triceps. By bringing your hands closer together on the bar, you shift more of the workload from the chest to the triceps, helping to build pressing power.
- **Overhead Triceps Extension**: Using a dumbbell or resistance band, perform overhead triceps extensions to target the long head of the triceps. This exercise helps to improve lockout strength during the bench press, particularly during the final phase of the lift.
- **Skull Crushers (Lying Triceps Extensions)**: Lying on a bench, hold a barbell or dumbbells with your arms extended above you. Lower the weights toward your forehead by bending your elbows, and then press them back up. This exercise isolates the triceps and enhances lockout strength, making it an excellent accessory for improving the bench press.

5. Pec and Shoulder Activation

Before you attempt a heavy set of bench presses, it's important to activate the chest and shoulder muscles to ensure optimal performance and reduce the risk of injury. The following exercises can help prime these muscle groups for the lift:

- **Chest Flyes**: Using dumbbells or a cable machine, perform chest flyes to activate the pecs and prepare them for pressing. The wide range of motion in this exercise helps warm up the muscles and improves their activation during the bench press.
- **Incline Dumbbell Presses**: The incline dumbbell press targets the upper chest and shoulders, complementing the flat bench press. By strengthening the upper part of the chest, you create a more balanced pressing motion, leading to improved overall performance.
- **Band Push-Ups**: Adding a resistance band to push-ups increases the difficulty and activates the chest, shoulders, and triceps in a way that mirrors the bench press. The added resistance forces your muscles to work harder, improving endurance and strength for the bench press.

Conclusion

Accessory movements for the bench press are a crucial component of any strength training program. By incorporating exercises that target the rotator cuff, improve shoulder mobility, strengthen stabilizing muscles, and enhance triceps power, you can improve your bench press performance while reducing the risk of injury. Consistent work on these accessory exercises will help you unlock new levels of strength and build a more balanced, resilient upper body. As you progress in your training, these exercises will not only support your bench press but will also contribute to your overall functional strength and performance.

Chapter 9: Overcoming Plateaus in the Bench Press

As you progress in your strength training journey, it's inevitable that you will encounter periods where your bench press progress stalls. These plateaus can be frustrating, but they are a natural part of the training process. Overcoming plateaus is an essential skill for every lifter, and with the right strategies, you can push through them and continue to see gains. In this chapter, we will explore how to identify plateaus, adjust your training program, utilize periodization and tempo variations, and employ mental strategies to break through your limits.

1. Identifying Strength Plateaus

Before diving into solutions, it's important to first understand what constitutes a plateau and how to recognize when you're stuck. A plateau occurs when your performance in a specific lift—like the bench press—stagnates, despite consistent effort and progressive overload. Key indicators of a plateau include:

- **Failure to Increase Weights**: If you've been consistently trying to add weight to the bar but can no longer achieve even small increments, you may have hit a plateau.
- **Diminishing Reps**: If your reps or sets are dropping off or you're unable to maintain previous volume at the same weight, it could be a sign that your body is no longer adapting to the training stimulus.
- **Feeling Stagnant**: A lack of motivation, persistent fatigue, or feelings of frustration can indicate that you're no longer experiencing the same level of progress. Training becomes more mentally taxing, and recovery takes longer.

Identifying a plateau early on allows you to take corrective action before it severely hampers your long-term progress.

2. Adjusting the Program

The first step to overcoming a plateau is to change your training approach. Constantly doing the same exercises, rep schemes, and intensities can lead to adaptation, where the body no longer responds to the stimulus in a productive way. Here are a few strategies for breaking through that plateau:

- **Change Your Rep Scheme**: The bench press can be trained effectively with a variety of rep schemes, including low reps (1-5) for strength, moderate reps (6-10) for hypertrophy, and higher reps (12-15) for endurance. If you've been stuck in a certain rep range for a while, shifting to a different rep scheme can reignite progress. For example, if you've been working in the 6-10 rep range, try dropping the weight and training in the 1-5 rep range with heavier loads for a few weeks. This can help you build maximal strength and activate different muscle fibers.

- **Increase Volume**: If you're consistently lifting heavy but not getting the volume necessary for growth, you may need to increase the number of sets or reps. Volume overload can stimulate further muscle growth and strength increases. For example, instead of doing 4 sets of 6 reps, increase to 5 or 6 sets of 8-10 reps. The additional volume will push your muscles to adapt and grow.

- **Change the Tempo**: Adjusting the tempo of your bench press reps can increase time under tension (TUT) and challenge your muscles in new ways. Instead of lifting with a standard 2-1-2 tempo (2 seconds up, 1 second pause, 2 seconds down), try a slower tempo, such as 4-1-4, to increase the intensity of the lift. The slower eccentric phase (lowering the bar) helps develop muscle control and may aid in overcoming sticking points during the lift.

- **Deloading**: If you've been pushing hard for several weeks, your body may need a break. Deloading involves reducing the intensity or volume of your workouts for a short period—usually one week—to allow your body to recover and reset. This can help break the cycle of stagnation and prevent overtraining.

3. Periodization

Periodization is a key concept in strength training that involves cycling through different phases of intensity and volume to prevent stagnation and optimize long-term progress. By structuring your training in cycles, you give your body time to recover and adapt, while progressively overloading the muscles. Here are the main types of periodization you can apply to your bench press training:

- **Linear Periodization**: This approach involves gradually increasing the intensity of your training while decreasing the volume. For example, you might start with higher volume (e.g., 4 sets of 8 reps) and progressively increase the load while reducing the reps (e.g., 4 sets of 5 reps, then 3 sets of 3 reps). Linear periodization is effective for beginners and intermediate lifters, as it provides steady and predictable progress.

- **Undulating Periodization**: This method alternates between different rep ranges and intensities on a weekly or even daily basis. For example, you might do a heavy day (1-3 reps), a moderate day (6-8 reps), and a light day (10-12 reps) within the same week. This approach provides variety, reduces monotony, and helps prevent plateaus by continuously challenging the muscles in different ways.

- **Conjugate Periodization**: This method combines strength, speed, and hypertrophy training by using different methods within the same week. For example, you could focus on maximal strength with lower reps and higher weights one day, then work on explosive power or speed with lighter weights and faster reps on another day. Conjugate periodization helps break through plateaus by targeting various aspects of strength and muscle development.

Each of these approaches can be tailored to your specific training goals and experience level, ensuring you keep progressing and breaking through plateaus in your bench press performance.

4. Mental Strategies to Push Past Limits

Overcoming plateaus isn't just about changing your workout routine; your mindset plays a huge role in pushing through tough moments in training. Here are some mental strategies to help you break through mental and physical barriers:

- **Visualization**: Visualization is a powerful technique used by top athletes. Before hitting the bench press, mentally rehearse the movement. Visualize yourself successfully pushing the barbell off your chest with perfect form and power. This helps build confidence and prepares you mentally for a successful lift.
- **Positive Self-Talk**: When you're struggling to progress, it's easy to fall into negative thinking patterns. Reframe your inner dialogue by focusing on your strengths. Tell yourself, "I am strong," or "I have the power to push through this." Positive affirmations help cultivate resilience and can make a big difference when attempting heavy lifts.
- **Set Mini Goals**: Instead of focusing solely on the end goal, set smaller, incremental targets along the way. For example, aim to add 2.5 kg (5 pounds) to each side of the bar every week, or try to add an extra rep to your sets. Breaking down big goals into smaller, achievable targets will help you stay motivated and make progress over time.
- **Train with a Partner**: Having a lifting partner can help you push past plateaus by offering motivation, encouragement, and assistance. A training partner can help spot you during heavy lifts, give you feedback on your form, and challenge you to push harder than you would on your own.

- **Embrace Failure**: While the idea of failing can be daunting, learning how to handle failure is essential for growth. Training to failure on certain sets or reps can be beneficial for developing mental toughness. It teaches you to push beyond your comfort zone and build resilience.

5. Incorporating Advanced Techniques

If you've been lifting for a while and have mastered the basics, you may need to incorporate more advanced techniques to break through plateaus. Some methods to consider include:

- **Training to Failure**: As previously mentioned, training to failure involves pushing yourself until you can no longer complete a full rep. While this can be physically taxing, it can stimulate muscle growth and break through strength plateaus when used strategically.
- **Accommodating Resistance**: Adding resistance bands or chains to your bench press is an effective way to increase resistance at the top of the movement, where you're the strongest. This helps increase power output and improves lockout strength. It's especially useful for athletes looking to develop maximal strength in their presses.
- **Board Presses and Floor Presses**: Both board presses (where a board is placed on the chest to limit range of motion) and floor presses (where you press from the floor to reduce the range of motion) are variations that target the lockout phase of the lift, where many lifters struggle. These variations help build triceps strength and break through plateaus.

Conclusion

Plateaus in the bench press are a natural part of any lifter's journey, but they don't have to be permanent. By recognizing the signs of a plateau early, adjusting your program with strategies like periodization, varying your training volume, tempo, and rep schemes, and utilizing mental tricks to push past limits, you can overcome these obstacles and continue to progress. Remember, strength building is a marathon, not a sprint. Embrace the challenge, stay consistent, and trust in your ability to break through every plateau.

Chapter 10: Advanced Bench Press Techniques

After mastering the fundamentals of the bench press, reaching the next level in strength training requires incorporating advanced techniques. These techniques go beyond the basics of form, reps, and weight and are designed to help you push past your current limitations, build even more strength, and enhance your pressing power. Whether you are a seasoned lifter or someone looking to break through a plateau, these advanced strategies can maximize your bench press potential.

In this chapter, we will explore some of the most effective advanced bench press techniques, including training to failure, accommodating resistance using bands and chains, and various bench press variations like board presses and floor presses. With the right application, these techniques will add both strength and variety to your workout regimen, leading to greater long-term progress.

1. Training to Failure and Beyond

One of the most powerful methods for increasing strength and muscle hypertrophy is training to failure. This technique involves performing an exercise until you cannot complete another rep with good form. Training to failure recruits more muscle fibers, promotes greater muscle growth, and enhances the strength adaptations needed to break plateaus.

Why Training to Failure Works:

- **Maximal Effort:** Pushing your muscles to their absolute limit activates all muscle fibers, particularly the fast-twitch fibers, which are responsible for explosive strength.
- **Increased Time Under Tension:** Reaching failure extends the time your muscles are under tension, which is a critical factor for muscle growth.
- **Mental Toughness:** Training to failure builds mental fortitude, helping you push through discomfort and fatigue, which is essential for long-term progress.

How to Use Training to Failure:

- **Use sparingly:** While effective, training to failure can be taxing on the body and increase the risk of overtraining if used excessively. It's best to apply this technique in cycles, such as once every 2-4 weeks.
- **Progressive Overload:** Start with a weight you can safely press for 8-10 reps. As you progress, push yourself to failure with that weight, striving to increase the number of reps over time. Eventually, increase the load once you consistently hit failure with your current weight.

Key Considerations:

- **Spotter:** Always train to failure with a spotter, especially when attempting heavy weights, to ensure your safety.
- **Form and Control:** Even when pushing to failure, maintaining proper form is critical. Do not sacrifice form for extra reps, as this can lead to injury.

2. Accommodating Resistance: Bands and Chains

Accommodating resistance is a method used to increase the load during different phases of the lift. Unlike traditional lifting, where the resistance is constant throughout the movement, accommodating resistance (using bands or chains) changes the load depending on the position of the lift. This allows you to apply more resistance during the stronger portion of the lift (near lockout) and less resistance during the weaker portion (the bottom of the press).

Using Bands: Bands are typically attached to the barbell and anchored to the floor or the rack. As you press the bar upward, the bands stretch and increase the resistance. This is especially beneficial for improving the lockout portion of the bench press.

Using Chains: Chains work similarly to bands but provide a different feel. As you lift the barbell, more chains come off the ground, adding incremental weight to the lift. Chains are often used for strength-focused training, particularly in the lockout phase, and can be more forgiving than bands in terms of consistency.

Benefits of Accommodating Resistance:

- **Overcoming Sticking Points:** Bands and chains are particularly effective for strengthening weak points in your lift, especially when you struggle with the top portion of the bench press (the lockout).
- **Increased Power Output:** The gradual increase in resistance during the pressing phase helps improve power and speed, particularly beneficial for athletic performance and explosive strength.
- **Variety:** Adding bands or chains introduces variability to your training, preventing your body from adapting to the same stimulus over time.

How to Implement:

- **Start Slowly:** If you've never used bands or chains before, start with lighter resistance to get a feel for the change in loading. Gradually increase the resistance over time as you build strength and confidence.
- **Alternate With Conventional Training:** Use bands or chains in one of your weekly bench press sessions, while continuing your normal bench press program during other workouts to prevent overtraining.

3. Board Presses: Targeting the Lockout

Board presses are an excellent way to focus on the lockout phase of the bench press—the portion of the lift where many lifters fail. By using a board placed on your chest (or just above it), you reduce the range of motion and eliminate the need to press the bar through the entire movement, isolating the top portion of the press.

Why Board Presses Work:

- **Strengthens Lockout:** The lockout phase often requires maximal triceps and shoulder activation. Board presses help target and strengthen these muscle groups by removing the initial stretch reflex that occurs when the bar touches the chest.
- **Improves Confidence:** For those who struggle with the top portion of the bench press, board presses allow you to use heavier weights, boosting confidence when attempting a full bench press.

How to Do a Board Press:

- **Choose the Right Board Height:** Typically, boards come in different heights (2, 3, or 4 inches), and you can experiment with different heights depending on where you struggle most in the lift. A 2-inch board is ideal for targeting the mid-range, while a 3 or 4-inch board focuses on the lockout.
- **Set Up the Board:** Have a spotter place the board on your chest before you press. Lower the bar to the board, pause for a moment, and then press the bar back up.
- **Focus on Form:** Even though you're using a partial range of motion, maintain the same pressing mechanics as you would in a full bench press. Keep your back tight, elbows tucked, and focus on explosive force.

When to Use Board Presses:

- **Strength Focus:** Use board presses when you are looking to increase lockout strength or break through plateaus in the upper portion of the lift.
- **Periodization:** Incorporate them into a strength phase, such as after a few weeks of regular bench press training, to give your muscles a new challenge and increase triceps power.

4. Floor Presses: Engaging the Triceps and Shoulders

Floor presses are another variation that reduces the range of motion but places greater emphasis on the triceps and shoulders. Instead of performing the press from a bench, you lie flat on the floor, limiting the movement to the upper portion of the press.

Why Floor Presses Work:

- **Reduced Elbow Stress:** For individuals with shoulder issues or those looking to reduce strain on the elbows, floor presses can be a great option. The limited range of motion prevents overstretching and promotes shoulder health.
- **Triceps Activation:** With the bar starting from a lower position, the floor press emphasizes tricep strength in a way that regular bench pressing doesn't. This is ideal for improving overall pressing power and performance.

How to Perform the Floor Press:

- **Setup:** Lie on the floor and set the barbell up on the pins of a squat rack or have a spotter hand it to you. Your feet will remain flat on the floor, and your back should stay neutral, just as with a standard bench press.
- **Lower the Bar:** Slowly lower the bar until your upper arms are flat on the floor, keeping the elbows tucked. Ensure that your elbows don't flare out too much, as this could cause shoulder strain.
- **Press Back Up:** Press the bar upward with control, focusing on squeezing your triceps and chest as you reach the top. Engage your core throughout the movement.

When to Use Floor Presses:

- **Triceps Focus:** Use floor presses when you want to specifically target the triceps and shoulders. It is especially beneficial if you've reached a plateau in the top portion of the lift and need to strengthen the triceps for better lockout power.
- **Strength Cycles:** Incorporate them in cycles where your goal is maximal strength, particularly after several weeks of full-range bench pressing.

Conclusion

Mastering the bench press involves more than just learning the proper form and progressively adding weight. Advanced techniques like training to failure, using accommodating resistance, and incorporating variations like board and floor presses are essential for breaking through plateaus and continuing to build strength. By strategically integrating these techniques into your training program, you can target weak points, enhance power output, and push past the limits that previously held you back.

With consistent effort, focus, and smart application of these advanced strategies, you can elevate your bench press performance and take your strength to new heights.

Chapter 11: The Military Press: Overview and Benefits

The military press is a fundamental exercise that has long been associated with upper body strength and athletic performance. As one of the most effective movements for developing the shoulders, triceps, and upper chest, the military press is a staple in strength training programs worldwide. In this chapter, we'll delve into the anatomy of the military press, its key benefits, and how it contributes to overall strength development and functional fitness.

1. Anatomy of the Military Press

The military press primarily targets the **deltoid muscles**, which are located on the shoulders. The deltoids consist of three distinct parts:

- **Anterior Deltoid** (front): This part of the shoulder is heavily involved in pressing movements, especially when the arms are raised in front of the body.
- **Lateral Deltoid** (middle): The middle deltoid plays a crucial role in shoulder abduction (moving the arm away from the body) and stabilizing the shoulder during pressing movements.
- **Posterior Deltoid** (rear): Although less engaged in pressing movements, the posterior deltoid provides essential stability and balance to the shoulder joint during overhead presses.

In addition to the deltoids, the military press also works several other muscles:

- **Triceps**: The triceps are responsible for extending the elbow as you push the weight overhead.
- **Upper Chest (Pectoralis Major)**: Though not the primary muscle involved, the upper chest helps stabilize the barbell during the press and is particularly activated when the press is performed with a slight incline or a close grip.
- **Upper Back (Traps, Rhomboids, and Lats)**: These muscles help stabilize the shoulder girdle and assist in preventing excessive shoulder movement during the lift.
- **Core Muscles**: The military press requires a stable core for optimal performance. The abdominals, obliques, and lower back muscles are heavily engaged to provide balance and prevent excessive arching of the lower back.

2. Key Benefits of the Military Press

The military press offers a host of benefits that make it one of the best exercises for developing functional strength and enhancing athletic performance. Below are the key advantages of mastering this lift:

- **Shoulder Strength and Development**: The primary benefit of the military press is the development of shoulder strength and muscle mass. As a compound movement, it recruits multiple muscles and encourages balanced growth of the deltoids, particularly the anterior and lateral heads. Over time, the military press can significantly increase shoulder size and strength.
- **Upper Body Power**: In addition to building shoulder strength, the military press helps develop upper body power. The ability to press heavy weights overhead translates to improved performance in various athletic activities, including throwing, pushing, and lifting movements.
- **Functional Strength**: Unlike machine-based exercises, the military press mimics real-world movements such as lifting heavy objects overhead or pushing against resistance. This functional strength is crucial for daily activities and sports performance, making the military press essential for athletes and anyone seeking to improve their physical capabilities.
- **Core Stability**: The military press engages the core muscles, especially the obliques, rectus abdominis, and erector spinae. This creates a stable platform for pressing and helps improve overall posture and spinal alignment, reducing the risk of injury during other movements.

- **Increased Testosterone Production**: Compound lifts like the military press have been shown to increase testosterone levels, which is beneficial for muscle growth, fat loss, and overall performance. The military press, being a heavy, multi-joint lift, stimulates large amounts of muscle mass, leading to a greater release of anabolic hormones.
- **Improved Overhead Mobility**: Regular practice of the military press increases shoulder mobility and stability, which can improve performance in other lifts, such as the bench press and pull-up. It can also reduce the risk of shoulder injuries by strengthening the rotator cuff and increasing shoulder joint stability.

3. Military Press and Athletic Performance

The military press isn't just about building muscle; it has real-world applications in improving overall athletic performance. The lift contributes to the following areas:

- **Overhead Strength**: Whether it's throwing a football, lifting a barbell in Olympic weightlifting, or performing military-style tasks, overhead strength is essential. The military press improves your ability to generate power in overhead movements, enhancing performance in sports like basketball, volleyball, and swimming.
- **Postural Control**: Because of its emphasis on shoulder stability and core engagement, the military press helps athletes maintain good posture, which is essential for all sports. Proper posture improves breathing, balance, and the ability to produce force, all of which contribute to better athletic performance.
- **Injury Prevention**: The military press strengthens the shoulder and upper back muscles, which are vital for stabilizing the shoulder joint during explosive movements. By building strength and endurance in these muscles, you can protect the shoulders from common injuries, such as rotator cuff strains or shoulder impingements, which are common in sports like swimming and tennis.
- **Cross-Training Benefits**: The military press also complements other lifts such as the bench press, deadlift, and squat. By balancing pushing and pulling movements in your training, you can develop well-rounded strength, improving your overall power, posture, and coordination.

4. Mental Benefits of the Military Press

The military press is not only a physical challenge but also a mental one. Overcoming the psychological hurdles of pressing a heavy barbell overhead requires focus, determination, and discipline. Here are a few mental benefits associated with the military press:

- **Focus and Determination**: The military press demands total concentration, as you must maintain a strong, stable base while pressing the barbell overhead. With each lift, you train your mind to focus and push through discomfort, which translates into improved mental toughness in other areas of life.
- **Confidence Building**: Mastering the military press, especially when progressing to heavier weights, can be an empowering experience. The act of lifting substantial loads overhead builds confidence, not only in the gym but also in daily life. The mental toughness gained from overcoming a challenging lift can boost self-esteem and resilience.
- **Overcoming Limits**: As with other heavy compound lifts, the military press provides an opportunity to push past perceived limits. Each successful lift, whether it's hitting a new personal best or completing a challenging set, reinforces the idea that you are capable of more than you initially thought.

5. Integrating the Military Press into Your Program

While the military press is often considered a specialized lift, it should be a core component of any comprehensive strength training program. Whether your goal is to increase upper body power, improve athletic performance, or enhance overall strength, the military press provides numerous benefits that complement other exercises like the bench press and bent-over rows.

To maximize the effectiveness of the military press in your program:

- **Combine with Other Compound Lifts**: Integrate the military press with other fundamental lifts like the squat, deadlift, and bench press to create a balanced routine. The military press can be done on upper-body focused days, either at the start of the workout for strength development or after other pressing movements for accessory work.
- **Frequency**: For maximum strength gains, aim to train the military press at least once or twice a week, depending on your level of experience and recovery. This frequency allows you to build consistent progress without overtraining.
- **Progressive Overload**: As with any strength exercise, progressive overload is key. Gradually increase the weight, volume, or intensity of your military press over time to ensure continuous improvement. This will stimulate muscle growth and increase overall pressing strength.

Conclusion

The military press is a cornerstone movement in strength training that offers a wide range of physical, functional, and mental benefits. It develops the shoulders, enhances upper body power, and improves overall athleticism. Whether you are an athlete, a bodybuilder, or someone looking to increase general strength and functionality, incorporating the military press into your training routine is essential. By mastering this lift, you'll build a strong foundation for total body strength, improve athletic performance, and develop the mental fortitude to push past your limits.

Chapter 12: Perfecting Your Form

The military press is one of the most effective upper body exercises for building strength, power, and shoulder stability. However, mastering the technique is essential not only for maximizing performance but also for preventing injury. In this chapter, we will break down the perfect form for the military press, focusing on the key elements of posture, core engagement, and pressing strategy to ensure you are pressing safely and effectively.

1. Setting Up for Success

A strong military press begins with a solid setup. Ensuring your body is positioned correctly from the start will lay the foundation for a safe and efficient lift.

- **Foot Position**: Start by standing with your feet shoulder-width apart, firmly planted on the floor. Your toes should be pointing straight ahead or slightly outward. This stable base allows you to engage your legs and core during the lift, contributing to better overall power and stability. Keep your feet flat, pressing them into the floor to maintain balance throughout the movement.
- **Grip**: The grip should be just outside shoulder width. When gripping the bar, your wrists should be straight—not bent back—so that the bar rests comfortably in your palms. A false grip (thumbs around the bar) or a regular grip (thumbs wrapped around) can both work, but ensure that your wrists remain aligned and stable throughout the lift.
- **Bar Placement**: The bar should rest just above your clavicles when starting the lift. This position ensures that the bar is in the most efficient place to press upward without excessive strain on the shoulders. If the bar is too high on your chest or too low, you'll struggle to press effectively.
- **Engaging Your Core**: Before you begin the press, take a deep breath and brace your core. This is crucial for maintaining stability during the lift. Imagine trying to push your belly button into your spine as you tighten your abdominals and lower back muscles. A strong core prevents excessive arching in the lower back and ensures that the force you generate from your legs and torso is transferred efficiently through your arms.

- **Scapular Retraction**: Pull your shoulder blades back and down (as if trying to pinch a pencil between them). This posture helps to stabilize the shoulder joint and reduces the risk of shoulder impingement or strain during the press. Keeping your shoulders retracted will also allow for a stronger, more controlled movement.

2. The Pressing Movement

Now that you're set up with the right position, let's break down the pressing motion itself. Mastering the technique is key to both lifting heavier and maintaining long-term joint health.

- **Initiate with the Legs**: Although the military press is an upper-body movement, the legs play a significant role in stabilizing your body during the lift. Before you begin the press, engage your glutes and quads by pushing your feet into the floor. This helps lock your body into place and prepares you for a strong lift.

- **Pressing the Bar**: Begin by pressing the barbell directly overhead in a straight line. The bar should follow a vertical path, not drifting forward or backward. As you press, your elbows should move from a slightly forward position to fully locked out above the shoulders. Avoid flaring your elbows too much, as this can place unnecessary strain on the shoulders.

- **Head and Neck Position**: As you press the bar up, it's important to slightly move your head back to allow the bar to pass directly over your face. Once the bar is past your forehead, your head should return to a neutral position. Keeping your head aligned with your spine helps maintain a strong base of support while preventing unnecessary tension in the neck.

- **Full Extension**: At the top of the press, your arms should be fully extended with your elbows locked out. At this point, your shoulders, elbows, and wrists should form a straight line. The bar should be stacked directly over your body to maintain the best mechanical advantage. Avoid leaning back or excessively arching your back at the top of the press. Keeping a neutral spine is crucial for minimizing the risk of injury.

3. The Descent and Reset

After reaching the top of the press, you must carefully control the bar as you lower it. While it may be tempting to let the bar drop, maintaining control over the descent is vital for both safety and muscle engagement.

- **Controlled Descent**: Lower the bar slowly and with control, keeping the same path as when pressing upward. Resist the urge to let gravity take over. A slow, controlled descent increases time under tension and provides an additional strength-building benefit. Aim for about a 3-4 second lowering phase to maximize muscle engagement in the shoulders and triceps.
- **Breathing**: As you lower the bar, exhale slowly and ensure you are maintaining tension in your core. You can take another deep breath at the bottom of the movement to brace yourself before initiating the next rep. Keep a consistent breathing pattern throughout the lift to maintain stability and power.
- **Repetitions and Pauses**: For optimal strength gains, it's important to decide whether you want to train for maximal strength or hypertrophy. If your goal is strength, consider performing each rep with minimal rest at the bottom and focusing on quick, explosive movements. If your goal is hypertrophy or endurance, you may want to incorporate a brief pause at the bottom of each rep, ensuring your muscles are under constant tension for a longer period.

4. Common Mistakes to Avoid

While the military press is a relatively simple movement, several common mistakes can hinder progress and increase the risk of injury. Here are a few to watch out for:

- **Arching the Lower Back**: One of the most common mistakes in the military press is over-arching the lower back to generate more power. This can cause strain on the spine and lead to long-term injury. Ensure that your core is engaged and that your lower back stays neutral throughout the movement.
- **Flaring the Elbows**: Letting your elbows flare out excessively during the press places undue stress on the shoulder joints. Keep your elbows close to your body and avoid excessive outward motion.
- **Not Using Full Range of Motion**: A common mistake is not lowering the bar to the chest or not fully extending the arms at the top of the movement. Both of these limit the potential for muscle growth and strength development. Be sure to use the full range of motion to activate all the muscle groups involved.
- **Allowing the Bar to Drift**: The bar should stay in a straight line overhead. Allowing the bar to drift forward or backward can negatively affect your shoulder health and decrease the effectiveness of the movement. Focus on keeping the bar over your body.

5. Pressing Strategies for Shoulder Health

The military press is an incredible exercise for building upper body strength, but it can also put significant strain on the shoulders if not executed properly. Here are some strategies to ensure shoulder health as you press:

- **Warm-Up Properly**: Before attempting heavy military press sets, it's essential to warm up the shoulder joint and surrounding muscles. Use dynamic stretches and mobility exercises, such as arm circles, shoulder dislocations with a resistance band, and light dumbbell presses to increase blood flow to the area and prepare for the heavy work ahead.
- **Shoulder Mobility**: A lack of shoulder mobility can limit your range of motion and lead to poor pressing technique. Incorporating mobility drills into your warm-up routine, such as external rotations, wall slides, and chest openers, can help improve your flexibility and range of motion for pressing exercises.
- **Rotator Cuff Health**: Regularly performing rotator cuff exercises can help strengthen the muscles that stabilize the shoulder joint. Movements like internal and external rotations with a resistance band or light dumbbells can help keep the rotator cuff healthy and reduce the risk of injury.
- **Overhead Press Variations**: While the military press is fantastic for building shoulder strength, incorporating other overhead pressing movements, such as dumbbell presses or incline presses, can help target different parts of the shoulder and reduce the risk of overuse injuries.

6. Conclusion

Mastering the military press is essential for building upper body strength, power, and functional movement. By focusing on proper setup, posture, and pressing technique, you can maximize your performance and reduce the risk of injury. Remember to engage your core, maintain a neutral spine, and keep the bar path straight to ensure an effective and safe press. With consistent practice and attention to form, you'll develop stronger, more resilient shoulders that will serve as a foundation for all your lifting endeavors.

Chapter 13: Accessory Movements for the Military Press

While the military press is a powerful exercise on its own, incorporating accessory movements into your routine can significantly enhance your shoulder strength, stability, and mobility. These supplementary exercises target the smaller muscle groups involved in pressing, improving your overall performance and helping to prevent injuries. In this chapter, we'll explore key accessory movements that will complement and strengthen your military press, focusing on rotator cuff exercises, scapular stability, triceps and deltoid strengthening, and essential shoulder mobility drills.

1. Rotator Cuff Exercises

The rotator cuff is a group of four small muscles that stabilize the shoulder joint, playing a critical role in preventing injury during pressing movements. Weakness or imbalances in these muscles can lead to shoulder pain, poor posture, and reduced pressing power. Strengthening the rotator cuff should be a priority for anyone who regularly performs the military press.

External Rotations

- *How to do it*: Attach a resistance band to a sturdy object at elbow height. Stand with your side to the attachment point and hold the band with your outside hand. Keep your elbow at a 90-degree angle and press your shoulder back. Rotate your arm outward, keeping your elbow pinned to your side, until your forearm is parallel to the ground. Return to the starting position with control.
- *Reps*: 3 sets of 10–12 reps per side.

Internal Rotations

- *How to do it*: Stand with your body facing the resistance band or cable attachment. Grasp the handle with the hand nearest to the attachment point. Keeping your elbow at 90 degrees, rotate your arm inward until your forearm is across your body. Slowly return to the starting position.
- *Reps*: 3 sets of 10-12 reps per side.

Prone Reverse Flyes

- *How to do it*: Lie face down on a bench, holding light dumbbells in each hand. With your arms extended straight below you, lift the dumbbells out to your sides, squeezing your shoulder blades together at the top. Lower back to the start position with control.
- *Reps*: 3 sets of 12-15 reps.

2. Scapular Stability Exercises

The scapula plays a vital role in overhead pressing, and poor scapular stability can limit your ability to press effectively. Strengthening the muscles around the scapula, such as the rhomboids, traps, and serratus anterior, will improve your pressing mechanics and help protect your shoulders.

Scapular Push-Ups

- *How to do it:* Start in a push-up position, with your hands directly under your shoulders. Without bending your elbows, squeeze your shoulder blades together, lowering your body slightly. Then, push your shoulder blades apart, raising your torso. This movement should come from your shoulder blades, not your arms.
- *Reps:* 3 sets of 12–15 reps.

Face Pulls

- *How to do it:* Set a rope attachment on a cable machine at face height. Grab the rope with both hands, and step back with your arms extended in front of you. Pull the rope towards your face, keeping your elbows high and wide. Focus on squeezing your shoulder blades together at the peak of the movement.
- *Reps:* 3 sets of 10–12 reps.

Wall Slides

- *How to do it:* Stand with your back against a wall, with your feet about 6 inches away. Press your lower back, upper back, and head into the wall. Place your arms in a "W" position, with elbows bent and forearms against the wall. Slowly slide your arms up the wall, maintaining contact between your arms and the wall. Lower back down with control.
- *Reps:* 3 sets of 8–10 reps.

3. Strengthening the Triceps

The triceps are responsible for locking out the military press at the top of the movement. Strong triceps not only help you push the barbell overhead but also reduce fatigue during high-rep pressing. Incorporating triceps-focused accessory exercises will help improve pressing endurance and strength.

Triceps Dips

- *How to do it*: Using parallel bars, support your body with your arms fully extended. Lower your body by bending your elbows to about 90 degrees, keeping your chest up and your body vertical. Push back up to the starting position.
- *Reps*: 3 sets of 8–12 reps.

Close-Grip Bench Press

- *How to do it*: Set up on the bench press as you normally would, but with your hands positioned about shoulder-width apart or slightly narrower. Lower the bar to your chest, keeping your elbows close to your body, then press back up.
- *Reps*: 3 sets of 5–8 reps.

Overhead Triceps Extension

- *How to do it*: Hold a dumbbell or a barbell overhead with both hands. Lower the weight behind your head by bending your elbows, keeping your upper arms close to your head. Press the weight back up to the starting position.
- *Reps*: 3 sets of 10-12 reps.

4. Deltoid Strengthening

Strong deltoids are essential for a powerful military press, as they bear the brunt of the load during the movement. Targeting all three heads of the deltoids—the anterior (front), lateral (middle), and posterior (rear)—will enhance your overall pressing strength and shoulder stability.

Lateral Raises

- *How to do it*: Stand with a dumbbell in each hand at your sides. With a slight bend in your elbows, raise your arms out to the sides until they are parallel to the ground. Lower back to the starting position with control.
- *Reps*: 3 sets of 12-15 reps.

Front Raises

- *How to do it*: Hold a dumbbell in each hand in front of your thighs. With a slight bend in the elbows, raise the dumbbells in front of you until your arms are parallel to the ground. Lower back to the starting position slowly.
- *Reps*: 3 sets of 10–12 reps.

Arnold Press

- *How to do it*: Hold a dumbbell in each hand in front of your shoulders, palms facing your body. As you press the dumbbells overhead, rotate your wrists so your palms face forward at the top of the movement. Reverse the motion as you lower the dumbbells back down.
- *Reps*: 3 sets of 8–10 reps.

5. Shoulder Mobility Drills

Maintaining adequate shoulder mobility is crucial for pressing exercises, especially the military press. Limited shoulder mobility can prevent you from achieving a proper range of motion and increase the risk of injury. Incorporating mobility drills into your routine will enhance your pressing performance and shoulder health.

Band Pull-Aparts

- *How to do it*: Hold a resistance band with both hands in front of you at shoulder height. Keep your arms straight and pull the band apart, squeezing your shoulder blades together. Slowly return to the starting position.
- *Reps*: 3 sets of 15-20 reps.

Shoulder Dislocations

- *How to do it*: Hold a resistance band or PVC pipe with a wide grip in front of your body. Slowly raise the band or pipe overhead, keeping your arms straight. Continue the movement behind your body,stretching your shoulders and chest. Reverse the motion to return to the starting position.
- *Reps*: 3 sets of 10-12 reps.

6. Conclusion

Incorporating accessory movements for the military press is essential for improving shoulder strength, stability, and mobility. By targeting the rotator cuff, enhancing scapular stability, strengthening the triceps and deltoids, and focusing on shoulder mobility, you'll build a more resilient and powerful pressing foundation. These exercises will help you overcome plateaus, prevent injury, and ultimately enhance your performance in the military press.

Chapter 14: Overcoming Plateaus in the Military Press

No matter how consistent and dedicated you are, it's inevitable: you'll hit a plateau at some point in your strength journey. The military press, with its demand on shoulder stability, triceps strength, and core engagement, can present unique challenges when progress seems to stall. This chapter will explore strategies to break through plateaus in the military press by utilizing deload phases, adjusting rep schemes, focusing on recovery, and targeting weak points in your lift.

1. Understanding Plateaus

A plateau occurs when you stop making progress despite continued effort. In the context of the military press, this may manifest as being unable to increase the weight lifted, or even feeling like your strength has regressed. There are several reasons plateaus happen, including:

- **Adaptation**: Your body has adapted to your current training routine, and your muscles no longer respond to the same stimuli.
- **Overtraining**: Insufficient rest, too much volume, or not enough recovery between sessions can cause fatigue to accumulate, leading to stagnation.
- **Weak Links**: A particular muscle or movement pattern may be limiting your ability to press heavier weights, such as weak triceps or poor scapular stability.

Breaking through these plateaus requires a combination of training modifications, recovery strategies, and mental toughness.

2. Deload Strategies

One of the most effective tools for overcoming a plateau is incorporating deload weeks into your training program. Deloading is a planned reduction in volume or intensity, allowing your body time to recover from accumulated stress and rebuild muscle fibers stronger. It's crucial to give your muscles a break to ensure long-term progress.

When to Deload

- Persistent soreness or joint pain
- A sudden decrease in performance
- Mental burnout or lack of motivation

How to Deload

- **Reducing Weight**: Lower the load to about 50-60% of your 1RM (one-rep max) and focus on maintaining form rather than pushing for new personal records.
- **Cutting Volume**: Reduce the number of sets or reps per exercise.
- **Lowering Frequency**: Instead of training the military press twice a week, reduce it to once, or incorporate lighter accessory exercises to maintain movement patterns without taxing the shoulders excessively.

Deloading allows the body to replenish energy stores, repair muscle fibers, and reset for future growth.

3. Adjusting Rep Schemes

Changing up your rep scheme can help shock your muscles into new growth, sparking further progress. If you've been following a standard 4x6 approach for a while, switching up your rep range can provide a fresh stimulus.

Low-Rep, High-Weight Training

Example

Higher-Rep, Moderate-Weight Training

Example

- **Pyramid Sets**: Gradually increasing weight while decreasing reps (e.g., 10 reps at 50%, 8 reps at 60%, 6 reps at 70%) can allow you to progressively overload while targeting different energy systems and muscle fibers.
- **Wave Loading**: In wave loading, you alternate between heavy, moderate, and light sets within a training cycle. For example, on one day, you may work in the 1-3 rep range, followed by a week with 4-6 reps, and then a light week with 8-10 reps. This variety will stimulate different muscle fibers and help overcome a plateau.

4. The Importance of Rest and Recovery

Rest and recovery are often overlooked but are crucial in overcoming plateaus. If you're constantly pushing hard without adequate recovery, your body won't have the chance to repair and grow stronger. Recovery plays a pivotal role in muscle adaptation, and neglecting it could be the main reason for your stagnation.

- **Sleep**: Ensure you're getting at least 7-9 hours of quality sleep per night. Sleep is when muscle repair and growth occur, and poor sleep quality can directly impair your performance in the gym.
- **Active Recovery**: Incorporating lighter activities like stretching, foam rolling, and mobility drills into your weekly routine will keep blood flowing to your muscles and improve joint health. Active recovery reduces muscle tightness and prevents overuse injuries.
- **Nutrition**: Adequate protein intake (roughly 1.6-2.2 grams per kilogram of body weight) is essential to support muscle recovery and repair. Ensure you're also getting enough carbohydrates to replenish glycogen stores and fats for hormonal health. A recovery meal post-workout that includes protein and carbs can help kickstart the repair process.

5. Variations to Target Weak Points in the Lift

Sometimes, the issue lies with specific weaknesses that hinder your press. Targeting these weak points with accessory movements can help improve your military press performance.

- **Triceps Strengthening**: If you struggle to lock out at the top of your press, your triceps may need more focus. Incorporate exercises like close-grip bench presses, dips, skull crushers, and overhead triceps extensions to build more pressing power.
- **Shoulder Mobility and Stability**: Limited range of motion or poor scapular control could be holding back your press. Incorporate shoulder mobility drills, band pull-aparts, face pulls, and scapular push-ups to enhance shoulder health and prevent compensatory movement patterns.
- **Core Stability**: A weak core can make it difficult to maintain an upright posture during the military press. Strengthen your core with exercises like planks, hanging leg raises, and ab wheel rollouts to maintain proper alignment while pressing overhead.
- **Explosiveness**: If your press lacks speed or you're struggling with heavier weights, incorporating explosive variations can help. Try push presses, where you use leg drive to initiate the lift, or even incorporate some Olympic lifts like the clean and press, which will train your ability to generate power quickly and efficiently.

6. Mental Strategies to Push Through Plateaus

Strength training is as much a mental challenge as it is a physical one. Mental toughness can be the difference between stagnation and progress, especially when facing a plateau.

- **Visualization**: Spend time visualizing your successful military press, from setting up to locking out the bar overhead. Visualizing success can help build confidence and reinforce proper form.
- **Goal Setting**: Break down your long-term goals into short, actionable steps. Focus on small wins, such as adding an extra rep or increasing the weight by 5 pounds. These small successes add up and can help push you through a plateau.
- **Mental Toughness Techniques**: When you feel the weight getting heavy, use mental cues to maintain focus and strength. Phrases like "drive through the floor" or "push the ceiling away" can help reinforce the movement and keep you focused on completing the rep.
- **Tracking Progress**: Keep a training log to track progress, even if the numbers aren't immediately increasing. Reviewing your progress can help you identify patterns, understand your training cycles, and give you the confidence to push through when you hit a wall.

7. Conclusion

Overcoming plateaus in the military press requires a multifaceted approach. By incorporating deload weeks, adjusting rep schemes, focusing on recovery, and targeting weak points, you can break through strength barriers and continue progressing in your training. Remember that plateaus are a natural part of the training process, and with the right adjustments, you'll come out stronger and more resilient. Keep pushing forward, and you'll soon find yourself pressing heavier weights with greater efficiency and control.

Chapter 15: Advanced Military Press Techniques

The military press is one of the foundational lifts for developing upper body strength, and once you've mastered its basic form, you can begin exploring advanced techniques to take your pressing power to the next level. These techniques will focus on maximizing your power, speed, and endurance, all while maintaining healthy shoulder mechanics and preventing injury. Whether you want to increase your 1-rep max or use the military press to enhance athletic performance, these advanced strategies will help you reach your goals.

1. Strict Press vs. Push Press vs. Jerk

While the military press is often referred to as a "strict press," there are variations of the movement that allow for greater weight to be lifted by utilizing the legs and hips. Understanding when and how to incorporate these variations can drastically improve your overall performance.

Strict Press (Overhead Press)

- *When to use it*: Use the strict press for building shoulder strength and stability. It's ideal for focusing on form, keeping the core engaged, and avoiding using momentum.
- *Key tip*: Focus on keeping your core tight and pressing the bar in a straight line. Any movement forward or backward in the bar path can cause you to lose efficiency and power.

Push Press

- *How to perform it:* Start with the barbell at shoulder height, engage your core, and dip slightly by bending your knees and hips. Then, explosively drive through your legs and hips, transferring the energy upwards to help press the bar overhead. Finish by locking your arms out at the top.
- *When to use it:* The push press is ideal for developing explosive power and improving strength endurance. It also helps you lift heavier loads than with a strict press, which can translate to increased muscle mass and strength in the upper body.
- *Key tip:* Focus on keeping the dip shallow—just enough to generate momentum—and ensure the bar travels in a straight line overhead to avoid unnecessary strain on the shoulders.

Jerk

- *How to perform it*: Start with the barbell at shoulder height. Dip down quickly by bending your knees and hips, then drive upward with your legs and aggressively "split" your stance into a front lunge while pressing the bar overhead. Catch the bar in the split position, then stand up to lock out your arms and feet simultaneously.
- *When to use it*: The jerk is perfect for maximizing your overhead lifting potential and improving your power output. It's especially beneficial for athletes who require explosive upper-body power, such as sprinters, football players, or crossfitters.
- *Key tip*: Focus on maintaining an explosive drive with the legs and a smooth transition between the dip and press. Your arms should remain straight during the split, and your catch should be controlled and stable.

2. Power and Speed Emphasis

Incorporating a focus on power and speed into your military press routine can help you break through strength plateaus and develop greater athletic performance. This is especially important for athletes who need to generate maximal force quickly—whether for sprinting, jumping, or combat sports.

Speed Work

- *How to do it*: Use about 50-70% of your 1-rep max and perform each repetition as explosively as possible. Rest only briefly between sets (around 45-60 seconds) to keep the intensity high.
- *When to use it*: Speed work is best utilized as part of a dynamic effort day within your weekly routine. This will increase power output, which is crucial for improving performance in both the press and other athletic movements.
- *Key tip*: Focus on perfecting the form during speed work. Moving the bar explosively with improper form can lead to injury, especially in the shoulders. Ensure the bar follows a straight vertical path to avoid unnecessary strain.

Paused Reps

- *How to do it*: Lower the bar to the chest or just below the chin, and pause for 1-2 seconds before pressing it upward. This eliminates the use of any bounce from the chest, forcing your muscles to initiate the press without relying on momentum.
- *When to use it*: Paused reps are excellent for improving lockout strength and for teaching better control during the press.
- *Key tip*: Keep your core tight and avoid sinking into a "lazy" position during the pause. The emphasis is on staying tight and bracing before pressing the barbell overhead.

3. Using the Military Press for Athletic Training

The military press is not just a strength-building exercise; it can be adapted to enhance performance in sports and other athletic activities. By using specific variations and focusing on the speed and explosiveness of the lift, you can improve functional strength that translates directly to your sport of choice.

Sport-Specific Emphasis

- For **sprinters**, emphasize explosive speed work, using lighter weights and quick, powerful reps to simulate the force needed for a fast start.
- For **football players**, use the push press to increase strength and power, which is essential for tackling, blocking, and pushing through opponents.
- For **athletes in combat sports**, such as MMA or boxing, focus on the strict press to improve shoulder endurance and core stability for throwing punches and clinching.

Olympic Weightlifting Integration

4. Programming Advanced Military Press Techniques

As you incorporate advanced techniques into your military press routine, it's important to properly program these variations to avoid overtraining and ensure continued progress.

- **Periodization**: Incorporating periodization into your training will allow you to cycle between different focuses such as strength, hypertrophy, and power. Plan your programming to include phases of strict pressing, push pressing, and jerking to continually challenge your muscles and avoid stagnation.
- **Combining Lifts**: On days where you focus on strength, emphasize the strict press with heavier weights. On power days, incorporate push presses or speed work with lighter loads. Keep jerk variations reserved for high-explosiveness days or after proper warm-ups to prevent injury.
- **Rest and Recovery**: Advanced lifting techniques can take a toll on the central nervous system (CNS). Ensure adequate rest and recovery between pressing sessions, particularly when incorporating heavy and explosive lifts. This will prevent burnout and support muscle recovery.

5. Conclusion

Mastering the advanced military press techniques—strict press, push press, and jerk—requires a solid foundation of technique and an understanding of how to develop power and speed. By strategically incorporating these variations, emphasizing speed and explosiveness, and adapting the press to fit your sport-specific needs, you'll not only improve your overhead strength but also enhance your overall athletic performance. Whether you're an athlete or a strength enthusiast, these advanced techniques will help you unlock new levels of power and efficiency in your training.

Chapter 16: The Bent-Over Row: Overview and Benefits

The bent-over row is one of the most effective compound exercises for developing the back and enhancing overall upper body strength. While often overshadowed by its pressing counterparts like the bench press and military press, the bent-over row plays a crucial role in achieving a balanced physique and strengthening muscles that are vital for both posture and performance in other lifts. In this chapter, we'll explore the anatomy of the bent-over row, its key benefits, and how it complements pressing exercises to help you build total body strength and improve overall power and performance.

1. Anatomy of the Bent-Over Row

The bent-over row is a horizontal pulling movement that primarily targets the muscles of the back, but it also recruits several other muscle groups. Understanding the anatomy involved will help you appreciate the full benefits of this powerful exercise.

Primary Muscles Targeted

- **Latissimus Dorsi (Lats)**: The largest muscles of the back that give the upper body its characteristic "V" shape. The lats are responsible for shoulder extension and adduction, making them key players in pulling movements.
- **Rhomboids**: Located between the shoulder blades, the rhomboids help retract the scapula and maintain shoulder stability. Strong rhomboids contribute to improved posture and a better ability to perform pressing exercises with proper form.
- **Trapezius (Traps)**: The traps are divided into upper, middle, and lower portions, each responsible for different movements of the scapula and shoulders. The middle traps are heavily engaged during the bent-over row, assisting with scapular retraction and maintaining shoulder integrity.

Secondary Muscles Involved

- **Biceps Brachii**: As with many pulling movements, the biceps play a significant role in the execution of the bent-over row. They are responsible for elbow flexion, helping to draw the weight towards the torso.
- **Rear Deltoids (Posterior Shoulders)**: The posterior deltoids assist in shoulder extension and stabilization during the row. A strong rear deltoid ensures that your shoulders remain stable and healthy during the movement.
- **Erector Spinae**: The muscles along the spine are engaged to stabilize the lower back during the bent-over row. Proper bracing and spinal alignment are crucial to protect the lower back and maintain proper form.

Core Muscles

The core plays a supportive role during the bent-over row by stabilizing the torso and preventing unwanted rotation. Engaging the abdominals, obliques, and lower back muscles helps maintain a strong, rigid position throughout the lift.

2. How Rows Complement Pressing Exercises

The bent-over row works in synergy with pressing exercises like the bench press and military press, ensuring that your training routine develops both the front and back of your body. While pressing movements primarily focus on the chest, shoulders, and triceps, the bent-over row targets the muscles that oppose these pressing motions—primarily the back and biceps.

- **Balancing Pushing and Pulling Movements**: Strengthening the muscles responsible for pulling is vital for maintaining balance in the body. Overemphasis on pressing exercises without corresponding pulling movements can lead to muscle imbalances, poor posture, and increased risk of injury. The bent-over row helps to correct this by promoting a more balanced, functional physique.
- **Improving Pressing Power**: A stronger back translates into more stability during pressing movements. The lats and rhomboids, when properly developed, contribute to shoulder stability and provide a strong base for pressing movements. When you row regularly, you're not only building a bigger back but also improving the ability to press heavier weights overhead or off your chest by providing better scapular stability.
- **Posture and Injury Prevention**: Rows can help counteract the effects of poor posture from prolonged sitting or from performing excessive pressing movements. By strengthening the posterior chain (the back, rear delts, and traps), you enhance your ability to maintain an upright, neutral spine during all lifts, reducing the likelihood of lower back and shoulder injuries.

3. Posture, Strength, and Hypertrophy Benefits

The bent-over row is a powerful exercise for developing strength, muscle mass, and overall athletic performance. Whether you're focused on building muscle or improving your functional strength, the row offers numerous benefits that will complement any training routine.

- **Posture Enhancement**: Modern lifestyles often lead to poor posture, with rounded shoulders and slouched spines becoming common issues. The bent-over row directly targets the muscles responsible for retracting the shoulder blades, which helps correct postural imbalances and promote a more upright stance. Strengthening these muscles encourages proper spinal alignment and reduces the risk of upper back and neck pain.
- **Strength Development**: By consistently incorporating the bent-over row into your routine, you build pulling strength that enhances overall upper body power. This translates to improved performance in other compound lifts, as well as everyday functional movements that require pulling, lifting, or carrying.
- **Hypertrophy (Muscle Growth)**: Rows are an excellent exercise for building muscle mass in the back. They provide an effective stimulus for hypertrophy by targeting multiple muscle groups simultaneously. When performed with proper form and progressively overloaded, the bent-over row can lead to significant gains in back size and density.

Tip for Hypertrophy

4. The Bent-Over Row in a Full-Body Strength Program

Including the bent-over row in your strength training routine helps ensure a well-rounded program that develops both the pushing and pulling muscles. The row complements other compound lifts like the bench press and squat by improving your overall strength, posture, and muscular endurance. Here's how to incorporate rows effectively into your program:

- **Row Frequency**: For optimal back development, include the bent-over row in your routine 1-2 times per week. Depending on your specific goals, you can program rows on upper-body pull days, alongside exercises like deadlifts, pull-ups, or lat pull-downs.
- **Variation**: There are several variations of the bent-over row, each targeting different parts of the back and providing a new stimulus for muscle growth. These include:

- **Barbell Bent-Over Row**: The classic variation that emphasizes overall back development.
- **Dumbbell Rows**: A unilateral exercise that targets each side of the back independently, helping to correct imbalances.
- **T-Bar Rows**: A great variation for building thickness in the mid-back.
- **Pendlay Rows**: A stricter, more explosive version that emphasizes power and strength.

Incorporating Rows with Pressing Exercises

5. Conclusion

The bent-over row is a cornerstone exercise for developing a strong, muscular back, and it complements pressing exercises by improving shoulder stability, posture, and overall upper body strength. Whether you're looking to improve your pressing power, correct postural imbalances, or simply add size to your back, the row is an indispensable part of a well-rounded strength training program. By understanding the anatomy involved, the benefits of the row, and how it complements pressing movements, you'll be better equipped to implement this exercise effectively in your training routine. Keep varying your row variations, focus on perfecting your form, and incorporate progressive overload to continually develop strength and muscle mass.

Chapter 17: Perfecting Your Form: The Bent-Over Row

The bent-over row is one of the most effective exercises for building a strong, powerful back. It's a staple in any serious strength training program, focusing on the development of the latissimus dorsi, traps, rhomboids, and rear deltoids. Mastering the form of the bent-over row is crucial, not just for maximizing muscle development but also for preventing injury and ensuring that you're getting the most out of the movement. In this chapter, we will break down every aspect of the bent-over row, from setup to execution, to help you perfect your form.

1. Setting Up for the Bent-Over Row

Before you even lift the barbell, it's essential to properly set up your body and the equipment. The bent-over row is a compound pulling movement that requires balance and coordination, as well as attention to detail in terms of body mechanics.

Foot Position

Key tip

- **Barbell Setup**: Position the barbell on the floor in front of you. Stand tall with your shins about 1-2 inches away from the bar. Bend down and grip the bar with a pronated (overhand) grip, with your hands roughly shoulder-width apart. Ensure that your grip is firm but relaxed, so you can focus on using your back muscles rather than your arms.
- **Hinge at the Hips**: With a slight bend in your knees, push your hips back (not down) while maintaining a neutral spine. The goal is to lower your torso at a 45-degree angle to the floor. The deeper you hinge, the more you'll engage the lats and rhomboids. A slight bend in the knees will help you maintain balance and allow your hips to travel back without rounding your lower back.

Key tip

Core Engagement

Key tip

2. Proper Back Angle and Posture

Maintaining the right posture throughout the bent-over row is essential to ensure the movement targets the correct muscles and minimizes the risk of injury.

Maintain a Flat Back

Key tip

Retract Your Shoulder Blades

Key tip

3. Grip and Arm Positioning

Your grip and arm positioning during the bent-over row are critical for targeting the correct muscles. While there are different variations of the row (such as underhand or neutral grip), the basic form remains similar across all versions.

Grip Choice

Key tip

Elbow Position

Key tip

4. The Pulling Phase: Breathing and Bracing

As you begin the row, it's important to focus on your breathing and the muscle engagement during the pulling phase. The pulling motion should be powerful but controlled, ensuring that you maintain tension in the target muscles throughout the movement.

Initiate the Pull

Key tip

Breathing

Key tip

Tempo

Key tip

5. Lowering the Bar: Eccentric Phase

The eccentric (lowering) phase of the row is just as important as the concentric (pulling) phase. This is where you can build muscle and strength by controlling the weight as you return to the starting position.

Controlled Descent

Key tip

Reset for Next Rep

6. Common Mistakes and Corrections

As with any exercise, there are common mistakes to avoid when performing the bent-over row. Correcting these mistakes will not only improve your results but also keep you safe from injury.

- **Rounding the Back**: This is the most dangerous mistake you can make when performing the bent-over row. It puts unnecessary strain on the lower back and can lead to serious injury. To fix this, always ensure that your back stays flat and your chest stays up during the lift.
- **Overusing the Arms**: If you rely too much on your arms to complete the row, you won't effectively target your back muscles. Instead, focus on pulling with your elbows and engaging your lats and rhomboids.
- **Jerking the Bar**: Jerking the bar to create momentum reduces the effectiveness of the row and can lead to injury. Always perform the row with controlled, deliberate movements.
- **Elbows Flaring Out**: Flaring your elbows out too much can shift the focus away from the lats and onto the shoulders. To correct this, keep the elbows close to your torso throughout the movement.

7. Conclusion

The bent-over row is a crucial lift for building a strong, muscular back. Mastering the form of the bent-over row ensures that you're getting the most out of the exercise while minimizing the risk of injury. By focusing on your setup, back angle, grip, and breathing, you can perfect the movement and make significant progress in your strength and muscle development. Consistently practicing proper form will help you unlock new levels of performance, whether you're a beginner or an experienced lifter.

Chapter 18: Accessory Movements for Bent-Over Rows

The bent-over row is one of the most effective compound movements for building a strong, balanced back. While the exercise primarily targets the latissimus dorsi (lats), rhomboids, and traps, it also recruits several other muscles that contribute to posture, grip strength, and overall pulling power. However, to maximize the benefits of the bent-over row and prevent muscular imbalances, it is essential to complement it with accessory exercises. These movements help to enhance the muscle groups engaged during the row, address weaknesses, and ensure balanced strength development across the entire body.

In this chapter, we'll explore a variety of accessory movements designed to build pulling power, improve muscle activation, and boost overall performance in the bent-over row. These exercises will strengthen the lats, rhomboids, traps, biceps, forearms, and more, providing a comprehensive approach to developing a well-rounded back and improving your rowing technique.

1. Lat Pulldown

The lat pulldown is an excellent accessory movement to reinforce the muscles used during the bent-over row, particularly the latissimus dorsi. This exercise mimics the pulling motion of a row but in a vertical plane, helping to build a stronger, wider back.

- **How to do it**: Sit at a lat pulldown machine with your knees under the pads. Grip the bar with a wide overhand grip, hands slightly wider than shoulder-width apart. Engage your core and pull the bar down towards your chest, focusing on using your lats rather than your arms. Control the bar as you return it to the starting position.
- **When to use it**: Include lat pulldowns in your accessory routine to develop lat strength and endurance. This movement is particularly useful if you struggle to engage your lats during the bent-over row.
- **Key tip**: Keep your chest proud and your scapula retracted throughout the movement. Avoid swinging or jerking the weight to ensure optimal engagement of the lats.

2. Face Pulls

Face pulls are a great accessory movement for improving the upper back, especially the rear deltoids, traps, and rhomboids. This exercise helps maintain good posture by strengthening the muscles that stabilize the shoulder joint and scapula. Face pulls also improve shoulder mobility and contribute to overall pulling power.

- **How to do it**: Attach a rope handle to a high pulley machine. Grip the rope with both hands, palms facing inward. Step back and pull the rope towards your face, keeping your elbows high and wide, and squeeze your shoulder blades together at the top. Slowly release the rope to the starting position with control.
- **When to use it**: Face pulls should be performed as part of your accessory routine to strengthen the upper back and improve posture. This movement complements the horizontal pulling of the bent-over row and helps balance out the work done by the pressing muscles.
- **Key tip**: Focus on retracting the scapula at the top of the movement to fully engage the traps and rhomboids. Avoid using too much weight, as this can compromise form and reduce the effectiveness of the exercise.

3. Barbell or Dumbbell Shrugs

Shrugs are an excellent accessory exercise for isolating the upper trapezius muscles, which play a key role in the finishing portion of the bent-over row. Strengthening the traps improves your ability to fully contract and stabilize your upper back during rowing motions.

- **How to do it**: Stand with a barbell or dumbbells at arm's length in front of you. Keep your arms straight, engage your core, and lift your shoulders towards your ears in a shrugging motion. Hold at the top for a second, then slowly lower the weights back to the starting position.
- **When to use it**: Shrugs can be used as part of your accessory routine to enhance the strength of the traps. Stronger traps can help with stabilizing the scapula during bent-over rows and other upper-body movements.
- **Key tip**: Keep your arms relaxed throughout the movement and avoid using your forearms to "pull" the weight. The movement should come entirely from your traps.

4. Single-Arm Dumbbell Row

The single-arm dumbbell row is a great variation of the bent-over row that targets the lats and rhomboids, while also emphasizing unilateral strength. This movement allows you to focus on each side individually, helping to correct any muscle imbalances that might affect your overall rowing technique.

- **How to do it**: Place one knee and hand on a bench for support, with the other foot flat on the floor. With a dumbbell in the free hand, row the weight towards your hip, keeping your elbow close to your body. Squeeze your shoulder blade at the top, then lower the dumbbell back to the starting position.
- **When to use it**: Incorporate single-arm dumbbell rows into your accessory routine to isolate the lats and address any asymmetries in strength between sides.
- **Key tip**: Avoid twisting your torso during the movement, and ensure the motion comes from your back muscles rather than relying on your arm to pull the weight.

5. Inverted Rows

Inverted rows are an excellent bodyweight movement for building pulling strength and improving the activation of the muscles targeted during bent-over rows. They work the entire back, including the lats, traps, rhomboids, and rear delts, and can be scaled based on your strength level.

- **How to do it**: Set up a barbell in a rack at waist height or use a suspension trainer (like TRX). Position your body under the bar, gripping it with both hands. Your body should be in a straight line from head to heels. Pull your chest towards the bar by squeezing your shoulder blades together, then lower yourself back down with control.
- **When to use it**: Inverted rows can serve as a great warm-up or accessory movement to reinforce proper pulling mechanics. They are also a fantastic option if you need to build the basic strength required for heavier rows.
- **Key tip**: Keep your body straight throughout the movement and focus on retracting your scapula. Avoid letting your hips sag or arching your lower back excessively.

6. Hammer Curls

While bent-over rows predominantly target the upper back, hammer curls are an effective accessory exercise to strengthen the forearms and biceps, which assist with grip strength during rowing movements. Stronger forearms and biceps will not only help you hold onto the bar but also improve the quality of your rows by allowing you to pull with greater force.

- **How to do it**: Hold a dumbbell in each hand with a neutral (palms facing in) grip. Keeping your elbows close to your body, curl the dumbbells towards your shoulders, then lower them slowly back to the starting position.
- **When to use it**: Include hammer curls in your accessory routine to improve forearm and bicep strength. These muscles play an important role in maintaining a secure grip during bent-over rows and other pulling exercises.
- **Key tip**: Focus on keeping your upper arms stationary and isolating the movement to your forearms. Don't swing your body or use momentum to lift the weights.

7. Key Flexibility Drills for Improving Range of Motion

Flexibility and mobility are key components of a well-rounded strength program. Improving your range of motion will allow you to execute bent-over rows with proper form, thereby reducing the risk of injury and maximizing muscle engagement.

- **Thoracic Spine Mobility**: Perform foam rolling or mobility drills to improve the flexibility of the thoracic spine (mid-back). This will allow for a better range of motion when retracting the scapula during the row.
- **Hip Flexor and Hamstring Stretching**: Tight hip flexors and hamstrings can limit your ability to properly hinge at the hips during the bent-over row, resulting in poor posture and less effective muscle activation. Incorporate hip stretches to improve your flexibility in these areas.
- **Shoulder Mobility**: Perform shoulder dislocations using a resistance band or broomstick to improve your range of motion in the shoulder joint, which will enhance your ability to perform rows with proper scapular retraction and depression.

Conclusion

Incorporating these accessory movements into your training routine will help to build a strong foundation for your bent-over rows, improving both strength and form. By targeting the lats, traps, rhomboids, biceps, forearms, and shoulders, you'll reinforce the muscles that play a critical role in rowing movements. Whether you're seeking to improve your overall pulling power, prevent imbalances, or increase hypertrophy in your upper body, these accessory exercises will help you achieve your goals and take your strength training to the next level.

Chapter 19: Overcoming Plateaus in the Bent-Over Row

Plateaus are a common hurdle in any strength training program, and the bent-over row is no exception. Whether you're a beginner or an advanced lifter, you will likely experience times when your progress stalls, and the gains you once made seem to plateau. This can be frustrating, but it's a natural part of the training process. Understanding how to identify, manage, and overcome plateaus in the bent-over row can help you break through these barriers and continue progressing toward your strength goals.

In this chapter, we'll explore various strategies for overcoming plateaus in the bent-over row. These strategies focus on adjusting volume, intensity, and exercise variations, as well as addressing any weaknesses or imbalances that may be limiting your progress. By employing these techniques, you can keep your rowing movements fresh, stimulating, and most importantly—effective.

1. Identifying Plateaus: What to Look For

Plateaus occur when the body no longer responds to the same stimulus, and muscle growth or strength gains stall. In the case of the bent-over row, signs that you're facing a plateau may include:

- **Stagnant Weight**: You're no longer able to increase the weight you're lifting, even though you feel you should be able to.
- **Decreased Reps**: You might notice that you're unable to perform the same number of repetitions at a given weight as you once could.
- **Lack of Progress in Assistance Movements**: Even though you're putting in the effort, accessory exercises and supplementary lifts such as lat pulldowns or face pulls are showing little to no improvement.
- **Mental Fatigue**: You may feel unmotivated or bored with your rowing sessions, and the excitement you once had for the exercise is gone.

Recognizing these signs early can help you adjust your training plan before the plateau becomes permanent.

2. Managing Volume and Intensity

One of the primary reasons plateaus happen is a lack of variation in training volume and intensity. Your body adapts to the stimuli you provide, so consistently doing the same number of sets and reps, or lifting the same amount of weight, can cause your progress to stall. To overcome this, consider implementing these changes:

- **Increase Volume Gradually**: If you've been doing the same amount of work for a while, try increasing your weekly volume. This can mean adding an extra set or increasing the number of repetitions per set. A gradual increase in volume can provide a new stimulus that challenges the muscles in a different way.
  Example: If you've been doing 4 sets of 8 reps, try 5 sets of 8-10 reps or increase your rep range to 12 per set for a few weeks.
- **Vary Intensity**: If your strength gains have stalled, it's time to adjust your intensity. This might mean lifting heavier weights for lower reps, or using lighter weights for higher reps, depending on your goal. Additionally, altering rest intervals or adding more explosive movements can help break through a plateau.
  Example: Incorporate low-rep, heavy sets (3-5 reps) for 3-4 sets in one session, and switch to moderate weights with higher reps (10-12 reps) in another session.
- **Change Tempo and Rest Periods**: Slowing down the eccentric (lowering) phase of the lift increases time under tension, which can lead to greater muscle growth. Alternatively, shortening your rest periods can challenge endurance and push the muscles to fatigue faster. Both approaches can reignite progress by adding new stimulus.

3. Targeting Weak Muscle Groups

Plateaus often occur because specific muscles involved in the bent-over row have become the limiting factor. Identifying and strengthening weak muscle groups can lead to improvements in your rowing performance and help break through the plateau.

- **Focus on Grip Strength**: A common limiting factor in the bent-over row is grip strength. If your hands tire before your back muscles, your performance will suffer. Incorporating exercises like dead hangs, farmer's walks, and wrist curls can help build a stronger grip.
  Tip: Use lifting straps if grip strength is a major limiting factor, but only as a temporary measure while you focus on improving grip strength over time.
- **Strengthen Your Lats**: Weak lats can limit your ability to properly execute a bent-over row. If you're struggling to engage your back muscles fully, consider adding lat-focused exercises like lat pulldowns, pull-ups, and single-arm dumbbell rows to your routine.
- **Improve Core Stability**: A weak core can cause you to lose form and limit your ability to generate force through the torso. Strengthening the core through exercises like planks, leg raises, and cable woodchoppers can help maintain stability and improve performance in the bent-over row.

4. Implementing Progressive Variations

One of the most effective ways to overcome a plateau is by changing the stimulus you provide to the muscles. For the bent-over row, this can be achieved through variations in form, grip, and positioning. These variations can target different aspects of the back and help break the stagnation in your progress.

- **T-Bar Rows**: This variation allows you to lift heavier weights and focus on the mid-back, particularly the rhomboids and traps. By incorporating T-bar rows into your routine, you can strengthen the pulling muscles and potentially overload them to break through plateaus.
- **Chest-Supported Rows**: A chest-supported row machine or bench isolates the back muscles by minimizing the involvement of other muscles such as the lower back and hamstrings. This variation can be particularly helpful if you're experiencing lower back fatigue during bent-over rows.
- **Single-Arm Dumbbell Rows**: Single-arm rows allow you to isolate each side of your back, which can help address any imbalances that may exist between your left and right sides. This can also provide a greater range of motion, which can enhance overall muscle development.
- **Pendlay Rows**: This variation involves pulling the bar from the floor with every rep, which helps to emphasize explosive power and lower back activation. Pendlay rows are a great way to introduce speed and power into your rowing movements, which can help break through plateaus.

5. Incorporating Deload Weeks

If you've been pushing hard for several weeks without seeing improvement, it may be time to introduce a deload week. A deload week involves reducing the intensity, volume, or both, to allow your body to recover and reset. This brief break can give your muscles and nervous system the chance to fully recover, leading to improved performance when you resume training.

How to Implement

6. Mental Strategies: Breaking Through the Mental Barrier

Sometimes, a plateau isn't just about physical adaptation but mental fatigue. Strength training can become monotonous, and the excitement of hitting new personal records can fade. To combat this, you can incorporate some mental strategies:

- **Visualization**: Imagine yourself executing the perfect bent-over row with good form and feeling strong. This mental practice can increase your confidence and help you push past mental barriers in the gym.
- **Goal Setting**: Reassess your goals and set both short-term and long-term objectives for your training. Breaking your progress into achievable steps can keep you motivated and focused.
- **Accountability**: Whether it's a training partner or a coach, having someone hold you accountable for your performance can help you stay on track and prevent you from becoming complacent.

Conclusion

Plateaus in strength training, especially in exercises like the bent-over row, are a natural part of the process. While they can be frustrating, they also present an opportunity to reevaluate your training strategies and make the necessary adjustments to continue progressing. By managing volume and intensity, addressing weak muscle groups, implementing variations, incorporating deload weeks, and using mental strategies, you can overcome plateaus and keep making progress toward your strength goals. Stay consistent, stay focused, and remember that breaking through plateaus is not just about lifting more weight—it's about smart training and continuous improvement.

Chapter 20: Advanced Bent-Over Row Techniques

The bent-over row is a foundational movement that targets the back, primarily working the latissimus dorsi, rhomboids, traps, and biceps. However, as you advance in strength training, simply performing the basic bent-over row may not provide enough stimulus to continue progressing. To break through plateaus, increase muscle mass, and enhance overall pulling power, it's essential to explore advanced row variations, targeting different angles and muscle groups. In this chapter, we'll explore several advanced techniques to take your bent-over row to the next level, ensuring balanced back development and improved pulling strength.

1. T-Bar Rows: Targeting the Mid and Upper Back

T-Bar rows are an advanced variation that isolates the mid-back and traps while allowing you to lift heavier weights compared to the standard barbell row. This exercise emphasizes horizontal pulling and helps to build thickness and power in the back, especially the rhomboids and middle traps.

- **How to do it**: Set up a T-Bar row machine or landmine attachment. Position yourself with your feet shoulder-width apart and knees slightly bent. Grip the handles or bar with a pronated (overhand) grip and pull the weight towards your torso, keeping your elbows close to your body. Focus on retracting your shoulder blades at the top of the movement and squeezing your mid-back.
- **When to use it**: T-Bar rows are excellent for building back thickness and targeting the rhomboids and traps. Incorporate them into your back training routine to vary the angle of your pulls and provide a new stimulus to your muscles.
- **Key tip**: Keep your back straight and avoid using momentum to pull the weight. The movement should come from your back muscles rather than your arms or lower back.

2. Chest-Supported Rows: Reducing Lower Back Fatigue

Chest-supported rows are a variation that eliminates the need for lower back stabilization, allowing you to isolate the back muscles more effectively. This exercise helps to remove the strain on the lower back, which can be a limiting factor in the traditional bent-over row.

- **How to do it**: Set up a chest-supported row machine or use an incline bench to support your chest. Grip the handles or a barbell with a neutral or overhand grip. Pull the weight towards your chest while keeping your elbows close to your body. Squeeze your shoulder blades together at the top of the movement, then slowly lower the weight back to the starting position.
- **When to use it**: Chest-supported rows are useful when you want to isolate the upper back without compromising lower back stability. These can be a great option for lifters who struggle with maintaining proper posture during bent-over rows due to lower back fatigue.
- **Key tip**: Focus on keeping a controlled motion throughout the set. Don't allow your body to move or your chest to lift off the bench. Maintain a strong, steady pull using your back muscles.

3. Single-Arm Dumbbell Rows: Isolating Each Side for Balanced Strength

Single-arm dumbbell rows allow you to isolate each side of the back, which can help address muscle imbalances and improve unilateral strength. This movement also provides a greater range of motion compared to the traditional barbell row, allowing for a deeper stretch and contraction in the lats.

- **How to do it**: Place one knee and hand on a bench, creating a stable position. With the opposite hand, grab a dumbbell and row it towards your torso. Focus on driving the elbow back and squeezing the shoulder blade at the top of the movement. Lower the dumbbell with control and repeat for the desired number of reps.
- **When to use it**: Single-arm rows are excellent for targeting the lats and improving symmetry in the back. They're also ideal for lifters who experience difficulty engaging one side of their back during barbell rows.
- **Key tip**: Ensure that your torso remains stable throughout the movement. Avoid rotating your body or using momentum to lift the weight. The movement should come solely from your back muscles.

4. Barbell Rows from the Floor (Pendlay Rows)

Pendlay rows are a variation that emphasizes explosiveness and power by lifting the barbell from a dead stop on the floor with each repetition. This variation engages more of the posterior chain, including the lower back, hamstrings, and glutes, while building explosive strength in the lats and upper back.

- **How to do it**: Set the barbell on the floor with a loaded weight, and stand with your feet shoulder-width apart. Bend at the hips and knees to grip the bar with an overhand grip, slightly wider than shoulder-width. In one fluid motion, pull the bar explosively towards your chest, keeping your back flat and your core engaged. Lower the bar back to the floor, ensuring it comes to a complete stop before starting the next rep.
- **When to use it**: Pendlay rows are great for developing explosive pulling power, especially in athletes who need to improve their dynamic strength. They also help reinforce proper deadlift positioning and hip hinge mechanics.
- **Key tip**: Focus on driving through your heels and keeping your chest up throughout the movement. Avoid rounding your back, as this can increase the risk of injury.

5. Renegade Rows: Combining Core Stability with Upper-Body Strength

Renegade rows are a full-body movement that combines a plank with a rowing motion, requiring core stability and upper-body strength. This exercise is great for developing back strength while also engaging the core and improving coordination.

- **How to do it**: Start in a push-up position with a dumbbell in each hand. Row one dumbbell towards your torso while maintaining a stable plank position. Lower the dumbbell back to the floor and repeat on the other side. Make sure to engage your core throughout the movement to prevent your hips from rotating.
- **When to use it**: Renegade rows can be used as an accessory movement to improve core stability and back strength. They are also an excellent option for those looking to incorporate functional, compound movements into their workout.
- **Key tip**: Keep your body as still as possible while performing the row, avoiding any twisting or swaying of the hips. Engage your core to maintain a stable plank position.

6. Seated Cable Rows: Focusing on Back Width and Detail

Seated cable rows are a great accessory movement for adding variety to your rowing routine. By adjusting the grip and cable attachment, you can target different parts of the back and vary the stimulus placed on the muscles.

- **How to do it**: Sit at a cable row machine with your feet planted firmly and knees slightly bent. Grip the handle with a neutral or pronated grip, keeping your arms extended in front of you. Pull the handle towards your torso, focusing on squeezing the shoulder blades together. Keep your chest up and avoid leaning backward excessively during the movement.
- **When to use it**: Seated cable rows are excellent for targeting the lats and mid-back. By adjusting the grip, you can focus on different angles of the back for balanced development. They can be a great complement to your heavy bent-over rows.
- **Key tip**: Focus on pulling with your back muscles, not your arms. Keep the movement smooth and controlled, with a strong squeeze at the end of each repetition.

7. Integrating Rows with Other Pulling Exercises

To develop a truly powerful back, it's essential to integrate the bent-over row with other pulling exercises. These can include vertical pulling movements such as pull-ups and lat pulldowns, as well as horizontal pulling movements like chest-supported rows or face pulls. Combining different angles and types of pulls ensures balanced muscle development and improves overall back strength.

- **How to do it**: Incorporate a variety of pulling movements into your weekly routine. For example, pair bent-over rows with pull-ups or lat pulldowns for a balanced approach to building back strength. You can also alternate between different rowing variations throughout the week to prevent adaptation and promote muscle growth.
- **When to use it**: Use a combination of pulling exercises to ensure all areas of the back are targeted. This approach will lead to more comprehensive back development and enhanced pulling power.
- **Key tip**: Don't neglect accessory exercises like face pulls and rear delt work, as they play a crucial role in shoulder health and overall upper-body strength.

Conclusion

Advanced bent-over row techniques are essential for breaking through plateaus and continuing to develop back strength, hypertrophy, and overall pulling power. Whether you're targeting the mid-back with T-Bar rows, isolating one side with single-arm dumbbell rows, or adding explosive power with Pendlay rows, these variations will help keep your training dynamic and effective. By incorporating different angles, grips, and accessory exercises into your routine, you can maximize your back development and build a stronger, more powerful body. Keep experimenting with these advanced techniques to continually challenge yourself and push the boundaries of your strength.

Chapter 21: Designing a Complete Strength Training Program

Designing a strength training program that incorporates the bench press, military press, and bent-over rows is crucial for achieving balanced, total-body strength and performance. Whether you're a beginner or an advanced lifter, structuring a routine that combines compound lifts, accessory exercises, and adequate recovery is key to making consistent progress. In this chapter, we will explore how to create a comprehensive training program that targets all major muscle groups, ensures proper recovery, and allows for progressive overload to maximize strength gains.

1. Understanding the Importance of a Balanced Program

A well-rounded strength training program should consist of three main components:

- **Compound movements** like the bench press, military press, and bent-over row, which work multiple muscle groups simultaneously and form the foundation of strength training.
- **Accessory movements** to address muscle imbalances, improve joint health, and target secondary muscles that support the compound lifts.
- **Recovery** to ensure muscles repair and grow stronger after each session.

By combining these elements, you create a holistic program that not only develops strength but also promotes muscle growth, mobility, and injury prevention.

2. Structuring Your Weekly Plan

When structuring your training week, the goal is to balance the intensity, volume, and frequency of your workouts to avoid overtraining while ensuring continued progress. A typical program will feature 3-5 training days per week, with varying focuses to allow for muscle recovery and optimal performance.

Beginner Program (3 Days per Week)

- **Day 1:** Bench Press, Military Press, Bent-Over Rows, Accessory Chest and Shoulder Movements
- **Day 2:** Lower Body (Squats, Deadlifts, Lunges)
- **Day 3:** Bench Press, Military Press, Bent-Over Rows, Accessory Back and Arm Movements

Intermediate Program (4 Days per Week)

- **Day 1:** Upper Body (Bench Press, Military Press, Bent-Over Rows, Triceps, Shoulders)
- **Day 2:** Lower Body (Squats, Deadlifts, Hamstring Work)
- **Day 3:** Upper Body (Accessory Rows, Chest, Biceps, Core)
- **Day 4:** Lower Body (Lunges, Deadlifts, Glute and Calf Work)

Advanced Program (5 Days per Week)

- **Day 1:** Chest and Shoulders (Bench Press, Military Press, Chest Accessory)
- **Day 2:** Back and Biceps (Bent-Over Rows, Pull-Ups, Arm Movements)
- **Day 3:** Legs (Squats, Deadlifts, Leg Press)
- **Day 4:** Full Upper Body (Accessory Movements for Shoulders, Back, Chest)
- **Day 5:** Full Body or Specialization (Power Movements, Heavy Rows or Presses)

3. Combining Compound and Accessory Exercises

While the bench press, military press, and bent-over rows are the cornerstones of your program, it's essential to include accessory lifts that support these movements and enhance overall strength. These exercises help to improve stability, target secondary muscle groups, and correct muscle imbalances.

Accessory lifts for the bench press:

- **Triceps dips**: Focus on strengthening the triceps, which play a crucial role in the lockout phase of the bench press.
- **Chest flys**: Target the chest more directly, providing hypertrophy in the pectorals.
- **Shoulder stability exercises**: To help maintain shoulder health, exercises like face pulls and rotator cuff work are key.

Accessory lifts for the military press:

- **Lateral raises**: Strengthen the lateral deltoids, improving the overall shoulder structure and helping with pressing power.
- **Triceps extensions**: Focus on developing triceps strength, which is crucial for a strong lockout during the press.
- **Face pulls**: Strengthen the rear delts and improve shoulder health for pressing motions.

Accessory lifts for the bent-over row:

- **Lat pull-downs**: A vertical pull variation that targets the lats to complement horizontal pulling movements.
- **Single-arm dumbbell rows**: Work each side of the back independently to correct muscle imbalances.
- **Trap work**: Shrugs and upright rows can help strengthen the upper traps, which contribute to the stability of the shoulder girdle during rowing.

By combining these compound lifts with accessory movements, you'll not only enhance strength but also help prevent injury and imbalances that can result from focusing on the big lifts alone.

4. Frequency, Volume, and Intensity Recommendations

For optimal progress, it's essential to tailor your training based on your experience level. The following recommendations provide guidelines on frequency, volume, and intensity for each experience level.

Beginners

- **Frequency**: 3 training sessions per week
- **Volume**: 3-4 sets of 8-12 reps for most exercises
- **Intensity**: Start with light to moderate weight, focusing on form and technique
- **Rest**: 1-2 minutes between sets

Intermediate Lifters

- **Frequency**: 4 training sessions per week
- **Volume**: 4-5 sets of 5-8 reps for compound movements, 8-12 reps for accessory lifts
- **Intensity**: Use moderate to heavy weights (70-85% of 1RM)
- **Rest**: 2-3 minutes between sets for compound lifts, 1-2 minutes for accessory exercises

Advanced Lifters

- **Frequency**: 4-5 training sessions per week
- **Volume**: 4-6 sets of 3-6 reps for compound lifts, 6-12 reps for accessory movements
- **Intensity**: Train with heavy weights (85-95% of 1RM), using advanced techniques like drop sets and supersets
- **Rest**: 3-4 minutes between sets for compound lifts, 1-2 minutes for accessory lifts

5. Rest, Recovery, and Deloading Strategies

To achieve the best results, your body needs time to recover and adapt to the stresses placed upon it during training. Overtraining can lead to injuries and hinder progress, so incorporating rest and recovery into your program is essential.

- **Rest Days**: Schedule at least 1-2 rest days per week to allow your muscles to recover. On rest days, focus on light activity like walking, stretching, or yoga to promote blood circulation and flexibility.
- **Sleep**: Aim for 7-9 hours of quality sleep each night to ensure your body has the opportunity to repair and grow muscle tissue.
- **Deload Weeks**: Every 4-8 weeks, incorporate a deload week, where you reduce the intensity and volume of your workouts to allow the body to fully recover. This is particularly important for advanced lifters who often push the intensity and may risk burnout or injury.

During a deload week, you may reduce weights by 50-60% and lower the volume to 2-3 sets per exercise. Focus on technique and mobility work rather than pushing for new personal records.

6. Tracking Progress and Adjusting Your Program

Tracking your progress is essential for ensuring that you're continuously moving toward your goals. Keep a training log that includes the following:

- **Exercises performed**
- **Sets, reps, and weights used**
- **Rest intervals**
- **Notes on how you felt during the workout**

Review your progress weekly or monthly to assess improvements in strength, muscle growth, and performance. If you hit a plateau, adjust your routine by changing the rep ranges, switching accessory exercises, or focusing on improving form and technique.

Conclusion

Designing a comprehensive strength training program is the key to achieving total power and performance. By structuring your weekly routine around the bench press, military press, and bent-over rows, and complementing them with accessory movements, you can target all the major muscle groups, increase strength, and prevent imbalances. Incorporating proper recovery strategies and adjusting the program as needed will ensure long-term success. Remember, the journey of strength mastery is a marathon, not a sprint—consistency, patience, and progression are the cornerstones of achieving your goals.

Chapter 22: Nutrition for Strength and Performance

Strength training and proper nutrition are deeply interconnected. What you eat before, during, and after your workouts can significantly impact your performance, recovery, and overall muscle growth. This chapter will delve into the essential nutrients required for strength development, how to time your meals, and the role of hydration in supporting optimal performance. Whether you're a beginner or an advanced lifter, understanding how nutrition impacts your strength goals is essential for achieving total power and performance.

1. The Role of Protein, Carbohydrates, and Fats in Strength Training

To support muscle growth, repair, and performance, you need to provide your body with the right nutrients. Each macronutrient—protein, carbohydrates, and fats—plays a unique role in fueling your workouts and helping your body recover.

Protein: The Building Block of Muscle

- **Importance**: Protein is essential for muscle repair and growth. During strength training, muscle fibers undergo small tears, and protein helps to rebuild and strengthen them.
- **How Much Do You Need?**: The general recommendation for strength athletes is 1.6 to 2.2 grams of protein per kilogram of body weight (0.7-1 gram per pound). For example, a 180-pound (82 kg) individual would aim for about 130-180 grams of protein per day.
- **Sources**: Lean meats (chicken, turkey, lean beef), fish, eggs, dairy, legumes, and plant-based protein sources like tofu and tempeh are excellent choices.

Carbohydrates: Your Fuel Source

- **Importance**: Carbohydrates are the primary source of energy for high-intensity workouts. Without adequate carbs, your body will struggle to fuel your muscles, reducing your workout intensity and increasing fatigue.
- **How Much Do You Need?**: Carbohydrate needs vary depending on the volume and intensity of your training, but strength athletes should aim for about 3-7 grams of carbohydrates per kilogram of body weight, with more carbs needed on high-intensity training days.
- **Sources**: Whole grains (brown rice, oats, quinoa), fruits, vegetables, and legumes are great options that provide sustained energy.

Fats: Hormonal Health and Energy

- **Importance**: Healthy fats are crucial for maintaining hormonal balance, particularly for testosterone and growth hormone, which are vital for muscle growth. Fats also provide a slow-burning source of energy for long workouts or recovery periods.
- **How Much Do You Need?**: About 20-35% of your total daily caloric intake should come from fats, with an emphasis on unsaturated fats.
- **Sources**: Avocados, olive oil, nuts, seeds, fatty fish (salmon, mackerel), and coconut oil are excellent sources of healthy fats.

2. Meal Timing and Supplementation

What you eat and when you eat it can have a major impact on your performance, recovery, and muscle-building potential. Strategic meal timing ensures that your body has the necessary nutrients for energy and muscle repair when it needs them most.

Pre-Workout Nutrition: Fueling for Performance

- **Timing**: Consume a balanced meal 1-2 hours before your workout. This meal should include a mix of carbohydrates, protein, and a small amount of fats to provide steady energy.
- **Ideal Foods**: A piece of whole-grain toast with almond butter and banana, or oatmeal with protein powder, is an excellent choice.
- **Why It Matters**: Carbohydrates provide the energy needed for strength training, while protein ensures that muscles have amino acids available to prevent breakdown during the workout.

Post-Workout Nutrition: Maximizing Recovery

- **Timing**: Aim to eat a protein-rich meal within 30-60 minutes after training to kickstart muscle recovery. This is when your body is most receptive to nutrient uptake.
- **Ideal Foods**: A protein shake with a carb source (such as a banana or a piece of toast) is perfect for post-workout. Alternatively, a meal like grilled chicken with sweet potatoes and vegetables is another excellent option.
- **Why It Matters**: After lifting, muscles are in a catabolic state and need protein to rebuild. Carbs help replenish muscle glycogen stores, ensuring you're ready for your next workout.

General Meal Timing Tips

- Eat 4-6 smaller meals throughout the day to maintain energy levels and promote steady muscle growth.
- Stay consistent with meal timing to help regulate your body's nutrient absorption and muscle repair processes.

Supplements for Strength Training

- **Whey Protein**: A quick and easy way to meet your protein needs, especially post-workout.
- **Creatine**: One of the most researched supplements, creatine helps increase strength, improve power output, and reduce fatigue during high-intensity exercises.
- **Branched-Chain Amino Acids (BCAAs)**: These can reduce muscle soreness and help prevent muscle breakdown during prolonged or intense training sessions.
- **Beta-Alanine**: This supplement helps buffer lactic acid buildup, reducing fatigue during high-repetition or high-intensity workouts.
- **Fish Oil**: Omega-3 fatty acids help with joint health, reduce inflammation, and support overall recovery.

3. Hydration and Its Impact on Performance

Hydration is an often overlooked yet critical factor for strength training success. Dehydration can impair strength, endurance, and focus, leading to subpar performance and a higher risk of injury.

How Much Water Do You Need?

- A general guideline is to drink at least 3.7 liters (125 ounces) of water daily for men and 2.7 liters (91 ounces) for women. However, this can vary depending on climate, workout intensity, and body size.
- **Pre-Workout Hydration**: Drink 16-20 ounces of water 1-2 hours before training to ensure optimal hydration.
- **During Workout Hydration**: Aim to drink 7-10 ounces of water every 10-20 minutes during exercise, particularly in hot environments or during long sessions.
- **Post-Workout Hydration**: Replenish lost fluids with at least 16-24 ounces of water following exercise. Consider adding electrolytes to help restore sodium, potassium, and other vital minerals.

Electrolytes and Sports Drinks

Sports drinks or electrolyte tablets are particularly useful for endurance athletes but can also benefit strength athletes during prolonged sessions or intense workouts.

4. Special Considerations for Strength Athletes

While general nutrition principles apply to everyone, strength athletes have specific needs that should be considered to maximize performance and muscle development.

Caloric Surplus vs. Caloric Deficit

- **Building Muscle (Caloric Surplus)**: If your goal is to build muscle, you'll need to eat in a slight caloric surplus. This means consuming more calories than your body burns to support muscle growth and recovery.
- **Cutting Fat (Caloric Deficit)**: If you're focusing on fat loss while preserving strength, aim for a slight caloric deficit, making sure to maintain a high protein intake to prevent muscle loss.

Meal Composition Based on Training Days

- **Training Days**: On workout days, emphasize carbohydrate intake around your training window to ensure you have sufficient energy for your lifts and promote muscle recovery afterward.
- **Rest Days**: On non-training days, you may slightly reduce carbohydrate intake but maintain protein intake to preserve muscle mass.

5. Conclusion

Nutrition is a cornerstone of strength training success. By properly fueling your body with the right balance of protein, carbohydrates, fats, and hydration, you can maximize your strength, recovery, and performance. Strategic meal timing, supplementation, and adequate hydration are key to ensuring that your body has the energy and nutrients needed to power through your workouts and recover efficiently. With the right nutritional plan, you can optimize your training and take your strength to new heights.

Chapter 23: Recovery: The Key to Growth

In the pursuit of strength and performance, recovery is often the most overlooked component. Training hard and pushing yourself to lift heavier, perform more reps, or go for longer durations is essential, but without adequate recovery, all that effort can be wasted. This chapter will explore the vital role recovery plays in building strength and muscle mass, as well as effective strategies to help your body repair, grow, and prepare for your next session.

1. Sleep and Its Impact on Muscle Growth

Sleep is arguably the most important recovery tool you have, yet it is frequently neglected. Quality sleep is when your body undergoes the majority of its repair processes, including muscle growth and tissue regeneration. Without sufficient rest, your muscles cannot fully recover, and performance gains are diminished.

- **Muscle Recovery and Growth**: During deep sleep, growth hormone levels rise, stimulating muscle tissue repair and promoting protein synthesis. This is crucial after intense strength training, which causes microscopic tears in muscle fibers. Recovery allows these fibers to rebuild stronger and larger.
- **Sleep Duration**: Strength athletes should aim for 7-9 hours of sleep per night. Some individuals may require more sleep during heavy training cycles, while others might find 7 hours sufficient. Listening to your body's needs is key.
- **Sleep Quality**: It's not just about how much you sleep, but how well you sleep. Poor sleep quality can interfere with muscle recovery and leave you feeling fatigued during workouts. To improve sleep quality:

- Maintain a regular sleep schedule (even on weekends).
- Avoid caffeine, nicotine, and heavy meals close to bedtime.
- Create a cool, dark, and quiet sleep environment.
- Limit screen time before bed to enhance melatonin production.

Napping for Extra Recovery

2. Stretching, Foam Rolling, and Mobility Work

Although strength training is critical for building muscle, flexibility and mobility are essential for joint health and performance. Incorporating stretching and foam rolling into your recovery routine can reduce muscle tightness, improve flexibility, and prevent injury.

Stretching

- **Static Stretching**: Performed after workouts, static stretching involves holding a stretch for 20-30 seconds, targeting tight muscle groups to improve flexibility.
- **Dynamic Stretching**: Dynamic stretches, such as leg swings or arm circles, are best performed before workouts to warm up muscles and prepare them for the demands of lifting.

Foam Rolling

Focus on key areas such as the lower back, quads, hamstrings, and calves. Spend 1-2 minutes on each area, but avoid rolling directly over joints or bones.

Mobility Work

Incorporate mobility drills like hip openers, shoulder rotations, and ankle dorsiflexion into your recovery routine to maintain proper posture and prevent movement dysfunction.

3. Active Recovery and Low-Intensity Exercise

While complete rest days are important, active recovery can also aid in muscle repair. Low-intensity exercise boosts blood circulation, which accelerates the delivery of nutrients and removal of waste products from muscles, aiding in the recovery process.

Active Recovery Ideas

- **Light Cardio**: A brisk walk, light cycling, or swimming can stimulate circulation without putting stress on the muscles. Aim for 20-30 minutes of steady-state cardio at an easy pace.
- **Yoga**: Yoga improves flexibility, reduces muscle stiffness, and promotes relaxation. Many yoga poses, such as downward dog, child's pose, and cat-cow, are excellent for loosening up tight muscles.
- **Swimming**: Swimming is a great full-body exercise that promotes blood flow and provides low-impact movement for recovery, especially for individuals with joint or muscle pain.

Rest Days

4. Nutrition and Supplementation for Recovery

Nutrition plays an integral role in muscle repair and recovery. After strength training, your muscles need the right nutrients to rebuild and grow stronger. Ensuring proper post-workout nutrition is key to maximizing recovery.

- **Protein**: Consuming a protein-rich meal or shake within 30-60 minutes after a workout helps stimulate muscle protein synthesis and accelerate muscle repair. Aim for 20-40 grams of high-quality protein from sources like whey protein, chicken, turkey, fish, or plant-based protein powders.
- **Carbohydrates**: After a workout, muscle glycogen stores (the body's stored form of carbohydrate) are depleted. Eating carbohydrates after training helps replenish these stores, ensuring you have energy for your next session. Choose complex carbs such as sweet potatoes, quinoa, brown rice, and oats.
- **Healthy Fats**: Fats are important for overall recovery, especially for joint health and hormone production. Incorporate healthy fats like avocados, olive oil, nuts, and seeds into your meals.
- **Hydration**: Rehydrating after a workout is vital to restoring fluid balance, as dehydration can slow recovery. Drink water throughout the day, and consider a post-workout electrolyte drink to replace sodium, potassium, and other minerals lost in sweat.
- **Supplements for Recovery**:

- **BCAAs (Branched-Chain Amino Acids)**: BCAAs may help reduce muscle soreness and prevent muscle breakdown during recovery.
- **Creatine**: While primarily used to enhance performance, creatine also plays a role in muscle recovery by supporting ATP production during training.
- **Glutamine**: This amino acid helps with muscle recovery and immune function, particularly after intense workouts.
- **Fish Oil**: Omega-3 fatty acids from fish oil have anti-inflammatory properties, helping reduce muscle soreness and promote joint health.

5. Avoiding Overtraining and Preventing Injury

While it's crucial to push your limits in the gym, it's equally important to listen to your body and avoid overtraining. Overtraining occurs when the body does not have enough time to recover between sessions, which can lead to diminished performance, fatigue, and an increased risk of injury.

- **Signs of Overtraining**: These include persistent fatigue, irritability, difficulty sleeping, decreased performance, increased soreness, and a weakened immune system. If you experience any of these symptoms, it's essential to take a step back, reduce training intensity, and prioritize recovery.
- **Preventing Injury**: Proper recovery strategies help to prevent overuse injuries, which are common when training too hard without proper rest. Incorporate regular mobility work, stretching, and foam rolling to maintain flexibility and joint health. Always use proper form and technique during lifts to avoid strain on muscles and ligaments.

6. Conclusion

Recovery is where the magic happens. Strength gains don't occur while you're lifting weights—they occur during the recovery process. Adequate sleep, nutrition, stretching, foam rolling, and active recovery are essential components for muscle repair and growth. By prioritizing recovery and avoiding overtraining, you can improve performance, prevent injuries, and continue making progress toward your strength goals. Treat recovery as part of your training program, and you'll reap the benefits of enhanced performance, greater strength, and long-term success.

Chapter 24: Mental Toughness in Strength Training

Mental toughness is the often-overlooked ingredient that separates those who simply lift weights from those who truly build strength. The ability to push through physical discomfort, to maintain focus when your muscles are burning, and to continue striving for improvement when progress seems slow or plateaued is what defines a successful strength training journey. This chapter explores how to cultivate mental toughness and integrate it into your training regimen, ensuring that your mind and body are aligned for maximum strength development.

1. Building Resilience and Focus in the Gym

Training for strength is as much a mental challenge as it is a physical one. When you push your body to its limits, your mind plays a pivotal role in determining whether you succeed or fail. Developing resilience allows you to endure setbacks and stay focused on your long-term goals.

- **Resilience Through Repetition**: The process of strength training involves constant progression. At times, you may feel frustrated with slow gains or occasional setbacks. Resilience is developed by accepting these plateaus as a natural part of the process and pushing forward with a positive mindset. Each repetition is an opportunity to grow not only your muscles but also your ability to stay the course.
- **Focus Amid Discomfort**: Strength training is inherently uncomfortable, especially during heavy lifts. Your ability to focus during these moments is what can make or break your performance. The key to maintaining focus is anchoring your mind on the task at hand rather than the discomfort you may be feeling. Concentrating on your breathing, the movement pattern, and your posture can distract you from the pain and keep your body moving effectively.
- **Setting Micro-Goals**: Rather than focusing solely on the big picture, break down your larger goals into smaller, more achievable micro-goals. For example, if you're working to increase your bench press, set a micro-goal of adding 2.5kg to your lift every week. These smaller goals help maintain motivation and provide clear milestones for success.

2. Visualization Techniques and Setting Mental Goals

Visualization is a powerful mental technique that can enhance your performance in the gym. By mentally rehearsing a lift before performing it, you can prepare both your body and mind for the task ahead.

- **Visualization**: Close your eyes and mentally picture yourself performing the lift with perfect form. Visualize the movement in detail—from setting up your body to the path of the barbell and the muscles firing. This process helps create neural pathways that enhance your muscle memory and boost your confidence.
- **Positive Self-Talk**: Your internal dialogue has a significant impact on your performance. If you tell yourself "I can't do this," your body will often follow that suggestion. Alternatively, by adopting a positive mindset and using affirmations like "I am strong, I will push through," you reframe challenges as opportunities to demonstrate your strength.
- **Goal Setting**: Mental toughness thrives on clear and achievable goals. Start with a long-term vision (e.g., hitting a 200kg deadlift) and break it down into smaller, incremental goals (e.g., increasing your deadlift by 5kg every month). Set specific, measurable, achievable, relevant, and time-bound (SMART) goals, and track your progress.
- **Focus on the Process**: Rather than obsessing over the final outcome, embrace the journey of strength building. Focus on the work you're doing in the moment, whether it's your form, technique, or daily training efforts. A process-oriented mindset helps you stay motivated during tough times and reminds you that every session contributes to your overall success.

3. Strategies to Push Through Fatigue and Discomfort

Strength training pushes your body to its limits, and there will inevitably be times when fatigue sets in. The difference between a lifter who stops and one who keeps going often comes down to mental fortitude. Here are some strategies to push through those moments of discomfort:

- **The 5-Second Rule**: The moment you feel resistance—whether physical or mental—your mind may tell you to quit. Use the 5-second rule: when you feel yourself hesitate, count down from five and then act immediately. This can short-circuit hesitation and prevent you from talking yourself out of completing the lift.
- **The "One More Rep" Mentality**: Strength training requires you to push beyond comfort. If you're on your last set and your muscles are screaming, remind yourself to perform just one more rep. That "one more" mentality can often lead to breakthroughs, as it gets you to push past perceived limits and enter a new realm of strength.
- **Embrace the "Fight or Flight" Response**: When facing a tough set, your body will experience an increased heart rate, adrenaline release, and heightened awareness. These natural responses can be harnessed for better performance. Instead of seeing these physiological changes as signals to quit, embrace them as tools to boost your energy and increase your mental toughness.
- **Disassociation**: When you're deep into a tough set and the pain is overwhelming, it can help to disassociate from the discomfort. Focus on your form, your breathing, or the sound of the barbell moving in and out of its path. This mental trick allows you to push through the discomfort by redirecting your mind away from the pain.

4. Developing a Routine for Mental Resilience

Mental toughness is a skill that can be cultivated with practice, much like your physical strength. By establishing a routine that nurtures mental fortitude, you can train your mind to endure the challenges of strength training.

- **Pre-Workout Routine**: The mindset you bring into the gym can greatly impact your performance. Start each session with a mental warm-up, which could involve setting an intention for the workout, reviewing your goals, and doing a brief visualization of your lifts. By creating a consistent pre-workout ritual, you prime your mind for success.
- **Post-Workout Reflection**: After each session, take a few moments to reflect on what you did well and where you can improve. This reflection process helps you mentally process the session and solidifies your learning, while also reinforcing your growth. Use this time to focus on the progress you've made, no matter how small.
- **Resilience Training in Other Areas**: Mental toughness is not limited to the gym. Practice pushing through discomfort in other aspects of life—whether in work, relationships, or personal challenges. The more you practice resilience in various contexts, the stronger your mental toughness becomes.

5. Conclusion

Mental toughness is not something you are born with; it's a quality you can develop over time through consistent effort, practice, and commitment. By learning to manage discomfort, focus on your goals, and visualize success, you'll enhance your strength training experience and unlock your true potential. Developing resilience and mental focus will not only improve your performance in the gym but will carry over to all areas of life. So, the next time you're faced with a challenging set or a tough training day, remember: strength is as much a mental game as it is a physical one. Embrace the struggle, stay focused on the process, and watch your power and performance grow.

Chapter 25: Tracking Progress and Adjusting for Long-Term Success

Strength training is not just about lifting heavier weights or pushing yourself harder every session—it's about consistent, methodical progress over time. To achieve long-term success, you need to track your progress, assess what's working, and adapt your strategy accordingly. This chapter will guide you through the key components of tracking your strength gains, evaluating your progress, and adjusting your routine to continue improving year after year.

1. How to Monitor Your Strength Gains

Tracking your strength gains is essential for staying motivated, ensuring you're making progress, and identifying areas that need improvement. Without measurement, progress can be difficult to assess, and you risk stagnation or burnout. Here are some effective ways to monitor your progress:

- **Record Your Lifts**: Keep a workout journal or use a training app to log every session. Record the weight, sets, and reps for each of your core lifts—the bench press, military press, and bent-over rows—as well as any accessory movements. This will help you track incremental progress and make adjustments to your program.

- **Track Strength Gains Over Time**: In addition to tracking individual workouts, it's essential to assess your overall strength development on a broader scale. Take note of any increase in the maximum weight you can lift for a given exercise or the number of reps you can perform at a specific weight. Set periodic benchmarks to check your progress—e.g., monthly or quarterly.

- **Use Percentage-Based Progression**: Another method for tracking progress is percentage-based tracking. Start with a baseline (e.g., your 1-rep max or a moderate working weight) and track increases as a percentage. For example, if you bench press 100kg for 5 reps, and then later you bench 105kg for the same number of reps, you've made a 5% improvement.

- **Non-Strength Metrics**: Strength gains aren't just about how much you can lift; they also involve improvements in muscle mass, endurance, and recovery. Take regular body measurements and track weight, body fat percentage, and muscle circumference. This will provide a fuller picture of your progress and give you more data to fine-tune your program.

2. Adapting Your Routine as You Progress

As you make gains in your strength training, your body will adapt. Eventually, you may notice that your progress slows or even stalls. This is a natural part of the training process and is known as a "plateau." The key to overcoming plateaus and continuing to progress is knowing when and how to adjust your routine.

- **Increase Intensity**: One of the most effective ways to break through a plateau is to increase the intensity of your lifts. This could mean adding weight, increasing the number of sets or reps, or reducing rest periods between sets to increase training density. Always increase intensity gradually to avoid injury and maintain proper form.

- **Periodization**: Periodization is the practice of varying your training intensity and volume over time. You can divide your program into phases (e.g., strength, hypertrophy, power, recovery) to ensure you're always challenging your body in different ways. For example, after several weeks of heavy lifting, you might shift to a lighter phase that focuses on higher reps to build muscle endurance before returning to heavy, low-rep training.

- **Change Your Training Variables**: If you've been focusing on one rep range (e.g., 3–5 reps for strength), consider switching to a different rep scheme (e.g., 6–8 reps for hypertrophy or 10–12 for endurance). You could also modify other variables such as tempo, rest periods, or exercise variations to continue progressing.

- **Deloading**: Incorporating planned deloads into your routine is crucial for avoiding burnout and overtraining. A deload is a brief period (typically a week) where you reduce the intensity of your training by decreasing the weight, volume, or both. This allows your body to recover and come back stronger for the next phase of training.

- **Accessory Movements**: If you find that your progress in the bench press, military press, or bent-over row has plateaued, incorporating targeted accessory movements can help. For instance, if your bench press is stalling, you might add exercises that strengthen the triceps (e.g., skull crushers or tricep dips) or the shoulders (e.g., dumbbell shoulder press) to break through the sticking point.

3. Tips for Setting and Achieving New Goals Year After Year

The most successful strength athletes don't just set goals—they set goals that are challenging, measurable, and adaptable. As you make progress, it's important to recalibrate your goals regularly to ensure that you're always working toward something that will push you to improve. Here's how you can set and achieve new goals year after year:

- **Break Long-Term Goals into Short-Term Milestones**: Long-term goals are great for vision and motivation, but they can also feel overwhelming. To make them achievable, break them down into smaller, incremental milestones. For example, if your long-term goal is to bench press 150kg, break it down into monthly or quarterly targets (e.g., adding 5kg every month).

- **Set Performance and Process Goals**: Performance goals are outcome-based (e.g., hitting a new personal best), but process goals focus on improving the techniques, habits, and strategies that lead to performance success. For example, your performance goal might be to increase your 1-rep max in the military press, while your process goal could be improving your form, consistency in training, or nutrition habits.

- **Challenge Yourself with New Lifts and Variations**: In addition to improving your core lifts (bench press, military press, and bent-over rows), challenge yourself by adding new exercises or variations to your routine. These could include movements like incline bench press, overhead squats, or Romanian deadlifts. By diversifying your training, you keep things interesting and target muscles from different angles, enhancing overall strength development.

- **Celebrate Milestones and Reflect**: Celebrating milestones, no matter how small, is essential for maintaining motivation. Take the time to acknowledge your progress and reflect on how far you've come. At the same time, review your approach to see what worked and what didn't. Constant reflection is a powerful tool for fine-tuning your strategy and ensuring that you're always moving in the right direction.

4. Conclusion

Tracking your progress and adjusting your training routine is an ongoing process that evolves with your strength development. By consistently monitoring your lifts, reassessing your goals, and incorporating new training strategies, you ensure that your progress continues year after year. Remember, long-term success in strength training comes from being adaptable, patient, and willing to push through challenges. Whether you're a beginner just starting your journey or an experienced lifter striving for new heights, tracking your progress and adjusting your routine is the key to unlocking your full strength potential.

As you move forward, embrace the idea that success is not just about lifting more weight—it's about constantly improving, learning from setbacks, and setting your sights on new challenges. Strength mastery is a lifelong pursuit, and by applying the principles outlined in this book, you will be well on your way to achieving your goals and surpassing them, time and time again.

www.ingramcontent.com/pod-product-compliance
Lightning Source LLC
Chambersburg PA
CBHW082243220526
45469CB00009B/2861